THE TOPIC OF
CANCER

An inspired and practical guide that will help you take control when faced with Cancer.

JESSICA RICHARDS

Published by Jessica Richards in 2012
PO BOX 177, Sandy, SG19 2LL

email: jessica@jessicarichards.co.uk
website: www.jessicarichards.co.uk

A catalogue record for this book is available from the British Library

ISBN: 978-0-9570644-0-9

Printed and bound in the UK by Portland Print, Kettering.
Designed and typeset by b-created, St Albans.

In loving memory of my mother, Kathleen
b. 02.01.34   d. 10.07.09

And my father, 'Chuck'
b. 22.08.26   d. 08.08 10

I've included a couple of small photos at the beginning of each chapter. To me, their similarities in pattern, form and structure remind me that there has to be an underlying plan, a bigger picture. I find this idea very inspiring and I hope you do too.

Thanks to Mitch Murray for coming up with the title for this book.
Thanks to Karen Welman of Pearlfisher for the original cover design.

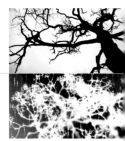

tree branches

neural network

Contents

Jessica Richards - Professional Profile

Jessica Richards specialises in personal transformation and leadership mentoring. Using her unique 'Changing the Groundhog Day' approach, (which breaks the patterns of self-limiting beliefs) developed over more than 25 years and thousands of hours of one-to-one sessions, she helps people achieve significant change in both their personal and professional lives.

In 2006, Jessica received an award for inspiring The Academy for Chief Executives at the 'Inspire' conference as well as the Founders' Award in 2009. Jessica is one of the most popular speakers in the history of the Academy.

Through her work with organisations such as Thomas International, Young Presidents' Organisation, The Academy for Chief Executives, and Vistage International as well as with top-level individuals, Jessica has facilitated rapid change through self-awareness which has enabled others to more consciously fulfil their personal and professional potential and therefore enjoy a more successful and meaningful life and business. For example, a senior manager in a publishing company came to see Jessica after being moved 'sideways' for the first time. Knowing there was no way up from there he sought a session with Jessica. He went on to become the President of that same organisation. An in-house lawyer of a well-known media company went on to set up his own specialist firm and is already leading the field with a very impressive client list and, at the same time, creating more balance and quality in his family life. The CEO of a major building company found the means to continue to grow his business success whilst creating more time with his wife and young family and is happier, healthier and even more successful for it.

Some of those who have benefited from Jessica's work include:

Dr. Maria Yapp
CEO of Xancam Ltd, a leading firm of business psychologists. Dr Yapp, was voted one of 2007's 'Top 100 Most Influential HR professionals'. This award is sponsored by Human Resources Magazine, the premier journal for senior HR decision makers in the UK.

Mark Addlestone
CEO of Beaverbrooks, the Jewellers which has, over the last three years come 2nd, 3rd and 4th in the Sunday Times 'Best Company to Work for' category. In each of those years Mark has come first in the 'Leadership' category.

Chris Oglesby
CEO of Bruntwood, sponsor of the Commonwealth Games in Manchester 2002.

Paul Lister
Multimillionaire conservationist whose Scottish estate, Alladale, is host to Jessica's annual spring retreat.

Steve Feery
Former CEO of C.O.I.N.S. International and founder of 'LIVESPACE' concept.

Martin Reed
Chairman and CEO of Thomas International, world leaders in business consulting.

Paul Ugo
CEO of Ugo Foods Ltd, which won 5th place in the Sunday Times 'Best Small Companies to work for 2007'.

As well as her work within organisations, or at her rooms in Harley Street, Jessica runs a number of seminars, either privately, or for organisations such as ACE Vistage CEO clubs and YPO. She also hosts an annual spring retreat in Scotland, a training programme which was hosted by ACE for its chairmen and members, and Wolf seminars on site at the Anglian Wolf Society where business and personnel issues are viewed from a completely different point of view.

Jessica has already helped hundreds of executives and community leaders meet their professional and personal goals.

All about me

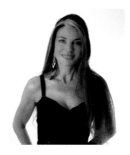

I was brought up in the 1950s and 60s, one of seven children. Our family experienced much hardship including spending a night in the police cells when our caravan (the family home) was almost afloat in a field during a flood. We were often on the move, which meant we had to change schools more times than you could shake a stick at! As the 'new kid' I was automatically put into the lowest class, but I worked my way up to being amongst the top three pupils in the top form. After a bout of teenage delinquency and a careers interview which consisted of, "and which factory are you going to work in?" I talked my way into Art College at the age of 16 where I trained as a pattern cutter and fashion designer and won a design prize from a sailing company for a design for sailing trousers that went into production.

Then I got a job in London as a pattern cutter at a leather couturier, which made outfits for film, and theatre as well as doing a robust trade in made-to-measure kinky stuff. I hitchhiked the ten miles to the station to get a train to London and did the same to get home on my return.

Eventually I moved to London after becoming a finalist in a modelling competition, but my modelling career was put on hold when at the age of 22 I became crippled with arthritis, a condition that had plagued me since my teens. After much hospital treatment my condition worsened until I was incapacitated from the neck down. Realising the treatment on offer wasn't likely to help in the longer term, I turned to a book my mother had given me, written by a doctor whose wife had suffered with arthritis. The doctor had devised a diet that completely reversed his wife's

condition. My deep interest in diet and natural healing made it an easy decision to stop all medication and go the diet route, which had an immediate effect and, over the course of the next year completely reversed my condition.

I became so well I took up martial arts, Karate first and then I trained as a Kung Fu instructor at a London Kung Fu school whilst at the same time resuming my modelling career until I was hit by a bout of pneumonia that left me bedridden for several weeks and housebound for some months afterwards. Weighing less than six stone I was unable to go straight back to modelling (in those days they preferred them blonde and curvy). One day, I was passing St James's Church in Piccadilly when I spotted a newly set-up market. I thought that if I could find the right product, a market stall might be the way to earn an income in the short term.

Shortly afterwards I was visiting my family, when a friend arrived who had a smoking pipe factory. I did the obvious and set up a stall selling pipes. I then found a London supplier and volunteered to work at the factory one day a week for free in return for being taught all there was to know about pipes. I expanded my enterprise to several stalls in London and due to popular demand, raised some funds from a bank to produce a mail order catalogue (which I designed myself) and set up my very successful mail order company.

During my time working on the stall, I met Gil Boyne, the man who was to offer me a scholarship to train as a hypnotherapist in the USA. When I got back to the UK, I immediately broke up with my partner (who'd become a heroin addict), sold my mail order company to the pipe factory owner and planned to move to the Isle of Man with my new partner. As a financial stopgap, so as not to use my capital, I took a job as a beauty consultant in Allders of Croydon. I knew I would need to set up some kind of a business on the Isle of Man, so I trained as a beauty therapist, taking over an empty unit next door to the main hairdressing salon at the main shop in Douglas. I had also secured two other jobs as fall backs, one working as a croupier in the Islands casino (a job I'd often fancied) and the other was as a martial arts instructor at the main sports centre.

Business went well for a couple of years, but then I had a return bout of a very severe eye condition which caused me to go completely blind in one eye. The surgeon recommended surgery which would give me a 50/50 chance of regaining my sight in that eye. I asked what my chances were without surgery and was told they were about the same. I decided that as my eye was already so painful from the condition and the steroids I'd endured being injected into my eyeball, I'd give surgery a miss for the time being and after devising my own eye exercises, gradually recovered my sight. During this time I realised my life just wasn't going where I wanted it to, and my relationship was coming to an end, so I sold up and returned to the States for further study and an internship. In order to learn more about hypnosis I put on stage shows both in the States and then back in the UK.

I set up my practice in London's Harley Street after meeting Marisa Peer, who already had a practice there. Marisa took me to Hertfordshire to look for somewhere for me and my two Great Danes which I'd brought from the Isle of Man. I noticed a clinic on my way back to the train station, and called in on the spot. I secured a room there for one day a week to supplement my London practice.

I built up both of my practices until I succumbed to another serious illness. I had uterine fibroids which almost caused me to bleed to death. I was rushed to hospital on the brink of cardiac failure, with apparently less than an hour to spare, clutching a letter to my chest forbidding a hysterectomy or any other surgery without my conscious written consent. The letter contained the details of my doctor and my lawyer and was signed by a witness. I was lucky to have a marvellous surgeon who was able to remove the fibroids by laser.

Living alone and running my business single-handedly meant that because of this latest illness, I had to start all over again. I began leading Chief Executive workshops, working live, and facilitating rapid change in people's lives and careers, using my highly effective 'Groundhog Day' process. I found myself in demand, both as a professional speaker and on a one-to-one basis amongst successful and influential CEOs at my Harley Street practice.

I was at the top of my game when in May 2007, I was diagnosed with breast cancer. I was told it was a relatively large tumour, up to 3.5cms, and advised that it would require 5 months of aggressive chemotherapy, a partial or total mastectomy, removal of my lymph nodes and radiotherapy followed by five years of drugs. I took control and after much questioning and visits to three hospitals, I decided to engage in an alternative treatment programme under medical supervision. Almost five years later, I am completely fit and well having used diet, intravenous Vitamin C, high doses of vitamins and minerals and most importantly, mental discipline.

I firmly believe that it's not the situation we are faced with which defines us but who we choose to be, in relationship to it. As my calling throughout my career has been to help others, it seems fitting and appropriate that I should write this book. It's a practical manual that can bring help and encouragement to people who are faced with a cancer diagnosis.

Introduction

As I write this in the spring of 2011, I am over four years on from a breast cancer diagnosis.

I know that a diagnosis of cancer or other serious illness can leave you feeling like you've broken down on a motorway alone and at night. Your only interest in that situation is to find a way to get your car back on the road and get home as quickly as possible. You would not be interested in reading up on the finer points of tow bars, or the technicalities of engine failure or perhaps someone else's harrowing account of what happened to them in a similar situation. All of these things may be of interest later, but for now, you feel you are in an emergency situation.

This is the reason I've written this ten-chapter emergency manual - to help you deal with the initial crisis and find your way home as soon as possible.

I am offering you a practical guide to help you remain calm and focussed in order that you can make rational and productive decisions in this most distressing of situations. I know exactly how you feel and although I can't physically be there with you on that particular road, through this book, I am there with you, every step of the way.

If you are reading this book because you want to help someone you know who has cancer, I aim to help you understand how it may feel from their point of view, and assist you in helping them in the most practical and beneficial ways. Having lost my mother to cancer, I know how helpless one can feel. To be honest, having had to deal with both situations, I personally found it easier to deal with my own illness than to worry about someone I love.

Throughout these pages, you will also read my own story, which I hope will bring you hope and optimism, bearing in mind that, I'm still not only alive but fit and well and leading a very full and normal life, having had no medical treatment whatsoever! I was recommended surgery, chemotherapy, radiation and drugs by three consultants at two different hospitals, but I chose an alternative route.

Many people who've heard my story say something like, "It's amazing what belief can do", or "I don't know if I could have the same amount of belief as you have in alternative treatment." I would like to make it very clear here that I did not base my treatment plan on belief. Belief had little to do with the decisions I made. I'm a rationalist. I view situations from a rational perspective. This is my nature, so when I was faced with a cancer diagnosis, I was able to be objective and look at it rationally including the possibility of falling off my perch. It's notable here that, although I chose a completely alternative pathway of care, I did it all under medical supervision. Even my alternative doctor, Dr Andre Young-Snell had spent twenty years working in the NHS.

It makes sense to me that when something becomes physical, we should seek the opinion and experience of a physician. This is what I did and was recommended a course of treatment, which I then proceeded to investigate given the barbarity of its nature and the risks involved.

Bearing in mind that my life would depend on the decisions I made, I rigorously asked questions and checked and re-checked all the facts and evidence and it was through diligently following through on every aspect that I came to the conclusion the treatment I was being offered simply did not add up as a reasonable choice for me at the time. The bottom line was, taking the conventional approach would have been a completely irrational decision based on the facts and evidence presented to me.

At the same time, I investigated the alternative treatments available, especially as I'd had some experience in this area at a hospital in Mexico about a decade before, where I'd seen terminal cancer patients returning for their yearly 'top up' treatments years after they were given weeks to live. In the meantime they were enjoying living normal lives. I decided on each part of my treatment in turn. I didn't just decide, 'right, I'm not doing any of that'. When weighing it all up it seemed clear to me that the alternative treatment, taking into account the facts and evidence, would provide me with the best chance of recovery and with no damaging side effects.

It wasn't that I totally believed in the treatment, I realised that much of it was down to my own attitude of mind. I'm as amazed as anyone else that I'm still here and extremely fit and well. It just seemed important to me that I should investigate the situation thoroughly and not make decisions based on fear and ignorance. I wanted the truth and the facts, not just to be pushed into things because they were all that was available and because that's what everybody else did.

Poignantly and tragically, nine months after my diagnosis, my mother was diagnosed with cancer. She passed away in July 2009. I can tell you that losing my mother to cancer was far harder than going through it myself. Nothing can change what happened to her or to other people I've seen lose their lives, however they chose to handle their illness. I offer this manual in order that other people don't have to accept anything purely on belief, but can base their decisions on facts and evidence, whether those decisions are in favour of conventional or alternative treatment, or a combination of the two. It may well be the case that I would have recovered anyway, but I've done so without feeling ill or damaging myself in any way - apart from my bank balance!

I'm not suggesting for a second that everyone should take an alternative approach. What I am saying is, do your due diligence, ask your own questions and make your own investigations in order that you can feel in control and confident in the knowledge that you've made informed choices for yourself. It's the best any of us can do. You owe yourself that much.

It is my sincerest wish and intention to present a balanced view and a practical guide, to give physicians, health care providers and patients a voice in order that together, we can develop the best possible relationships as we address our collective desire of returning to full health.

I have written this book so that you can feel safe and in control during your chosen pathway of care in the knowledge that you are in the safest of hands - your own. Remember, it's not the events in our lives that define who we are, but who we choose to be in relationship to those events.

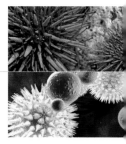

CHAPTER 1

I've been diagnosed with Cancer, where do I start?

Ten questions to ask yourself

1. To Tell or not to Tell.

On being told that you have cancer, one of the first things you will need to consider is who to tell. Really think about this one before it becomes common knowledge, as once it's out you can never close the door whereas you can tell more people as you go along.

The following is what I chose to do and the reasoning for it. But you must make your own call on this and do what feels right for you.

I chose to go to the recall screening alone (After a mammogram you will be recalled for further tests if abnormalities are found. Don't worry if this has happened to you as most prove to be a false alarm). I was pretty sure my result would be positive and I wanted to get my own head around it before dealing with anyone else's reactions. So, the question is, what happens when you've been diagnosed? Because you can't keep it entirely to yourself.

The first question I asked myself was not who should I tell but, who *needs* to know? This is a really important question. After the diagnosis, I chose to tell only on a 'need to know' basis. First, was my partner Alan, next, my close friend Astrid and a couple of my other neighbours who are also friends as I would possibly need to call on their help should I become incapacitated at any point. That was it on

the personal front. Next, I tackled the work front. I told only my secretary Olivia and the practice manager at my clinic in Harley Street. Then I told a few very close corporate colleagues as I valued their level-headed input as much as their friendship.

I asked everyone to keep it strictly confidential as, in the beginning, I didn't yet know the extent of the situation or which way it would go. I decided that, should the worst happen, I could at least continue with a relatively normal life (something every cancer patient craves) until the inevitable end. I did not want everyone to know too far in advance and for them to treat me any differently from normal or to have everyone on tenterhooks waiting for me to 'fall off my perch!' I kept it from my siblings and parents until after the results of the diagnostic lymph node surgery, when I had a plan and more of an idea of the prognosis. When I had this information, I still only told my parents. I needed to keep focussed on my plan and not have to deal with the fears of too many others.

I'd like to make a point here for those who are asked to be a confidante of a cancer patient. If you are, please remember that it is not your business to tell anyone else. I was dismayed to learn that someone I had trusted felt it was ok just to tell their best friend. Another person told someone else because they thought that person might find it helpful, even though it was very early days and I hadn't even told my family at the time. On another occasion, one of my close friends was told by someone who 'assumed they knew'.

Whatever you think and whatever you feel, please remember that it is not your call. Being asked not to tell means exactly that. Keep it shut!

2. Take their word for it or check it out yourself?

You may find that opinions differ from one consultant to the next so it's important that you investigate it thoroughly as it's not the exact science that many believe it is. Some may choose, as I did, to look into alternative and complementary options as well. The question for me was, should I just hand over my life to the medical profession or should I look into the situation as thoroughly as possible and base any decisions on facts found? Being a control freak, I couldn't possibly just hand everything over to a system, which, to my mind, becomes largely run by bureaucrats and administrators. My life could be at stake here and I didn't want to risk the chance of death due to a 'clerical error'. As you may have already guessed, I have a deep aversion to the element of admin in any area! My decision was partially influenced by an experience I'd had of spending time in

a Mexican hospital years before…. (Don't ask) Well, as you did ask, I was there because I was recovering from another serious illness (not cancer) and I went there for two reasons. One was to check it out as a possible place where I could refer my own clients who needed somewhere safe to convalesce and the other, for my own interest as I knew they specialised in alternative cancer treatments, something I'd long had an interest in. Upon arrival, I experienced breathing difficulties and ended up as an inpatient. It was here that I saw with my own eyes patients who'd years before been given only a few months or even weeks to live. They returned once a year for top-up treatments and check-ups and otherwise led completely normal lives!

It was quite funny really, I was with my friend Eldridge, a large black man in his sixties who suffered from sleep apnoea (a condition which causes the sufferer to stop breathing at frequent intervals during sleep causing them to awaken and therefore never enjoy the deep level of sleep necessary for normal functioning and wellbeing) and, because of the sleep deprivation it causes, he looked a lot more ill than I did. When the doctor came out, he went straight up to Eldridge, took his hands and said, "Come on my friend, let's see if we can help you." Eldridge was shocked and asked me later, "Do you think I look like a cancer patient?" I assured him that he didn't, he just looked more like one than I did!

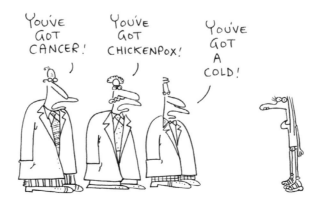

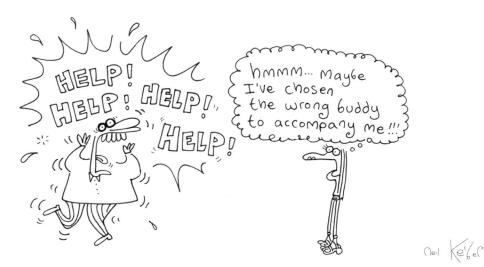

3. Choose your buddy.

Choose your partner or buddy to accompany you throughout the process. It's important to choose people who will support you without pressurising you to do things their way, and you definitely don't need people who panic or are negative by nature.

It's amazing how much time you have to spend taking care of other people emotionally. If you choose to go the alternative therapy route, don't be surprised or disappointed if your family are not included in this group. They may not share your views and through fear, are unable to be supportive in the way you need. It's quite common and often encouraged that you partner up with another cancer patient and go through the process together. Theoretically this makes perfect sense, but I experienced first-hand the devastating effect when my 'buddy' died. Even though we're aware this can be a possibility it doesn't soften the blow or the awful feeling of guilt I had when I spoke with her family. I know it may sound nuts but, I felt almost ashamed at being so well whereas she'd lost her life.

I had Alan and another close friend Marisa. Alan backed me totally whatever treatment I considered and he came to every consultant's appointment with me. In fact, my one enduring memory of Alan throughout this time is of him standing in the corner of various consulting rooms clutching my bra whilst consultants or radiologists were examining me.

Marisa had been a friend for many years and has written several successful books on self development and nutrition, so she was well equipped to support me. In fact, I arranged to stay with Marisa the night before the lymph node biopsy as she lived quite near the hospital. Alan was to meet us there later in the day to get me home. I was booked for surgery first thing in the morning as I suffer badly from the effects of anaesthetic and needed time to recover in order to leave that evening, as I was a day patient and had no intention of staying in overnight.

When we arrived, I got ready and Marisa assured me that she wouldn't leave my bedside, as I was paranoid about anyone administering any drugs whilst I was incapacitated. She'd brought herself a flask of coffee and I suggested that, as the bed was comfortable, whilst I was away she should have a lie on that and get some rest. She said that was a great idea as she would normally have a cup of coffee and read her paper in bed. I found out later there'd been a slight mix up and, after I'd been taken down to theatre, another team came for me. Seeing Marisa on my bed, they told her she was going down to theatre. Marisa began to protest and they said she should calm down and not worry, as she would be taken good care of. At this point a nurse popped her head around the curtain and exclaimed, "That's not Jessica Richards!" "What are you doing on her bed"? Marisa explained and got a telling off, as the nurse then had to change the linen in case of infection. I was relieved nonetheless, when I came back from theatre and, in my semi-conscious state, saw Alan and Marisa sitting there.

4. Which hospital do you want to be treated at?

Look into this carefully and don't be afraid to look at more than one if you don't feel comfortable with your first choice. You're probably going to be spending a lot of time there so it's important that you feel happy about their processes, accessibility and availability of treatment and facilities.

Before I was diagnosed I had never really appreciated the value of this choice, I'd always imagined I'd just go to the nearest hospital as I'd always done in the past. I had a chat with my GP who

CHOOSING THE RIGHT HOSPITAL:

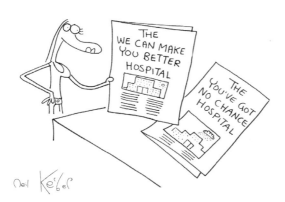

informed me of the local options. I didn't know how to make that choice. (I'd already had experience of most of the hospitals in my area, as I can be slightly accident-prone and no stranger to the A & E departments). I'd had a good experience of the first hospital my GP mentioned, but I also knew it was under threat of closure partly due to infection. The second hospital he talked about had several bad memories for me, and I told him, "I wouldn't take my dog there and he's been dead for seven years!" He laughed and said that it sounded like I'd already made up my mind. I then asked him which hospital he usually refers his breast cancer patients to. He told me, and added that it was a teaching hospital so there could be more treatments available should things not go well! I have to say that I eventually went to three different hospitals and chose the last one because of the consultant there. As I'd decided to go completely alternative at Dr Andre's clinic I asked to see the same consultant as one of his other patients. He'd monitored her through the same treatment as mine and at that time, she'd been clear for three and a half years. (She was diagnosed in 2002 and is still very much alive and well).

5. What are the practical things to be addressed?

If you haven't already done so you should make a Will and /or get your affairs in order. At the very least, it feels better to know that you've done this, so you can concentrate on getting well again. It also feels good to clear the decks of any unfinished business or outstanding official paperwork, so you have time to rest and not get stressed out about these things.

The first thing I did when I was diagnosed was to make a Will. I wasn't married to Alan and I wanted to make sure that, should I die, he wouldn't lose his home too. It was in the solicitors' office that I wished I'd attended to it earlier. I'm a 'doer' and, until then I'd just gone into action to deal with my health situation without any emotional fallout, but, as the solicitor left the room to get a witness and I sat there alone reading through my funeral arrangements and bequests, the gravity of the situation swept over me for a few seconds. However, I didn't allow it to take hold of me. When she returned I duly signed the documents and the cheque, which I joked she should cash whilst I was still around!

A few days later, I was crouching by my front door putting on my trainers before going for a run when the post fell through the letter box. I picked up my copy of the letter to my doctor from the hospital. I had to brace myself for this, as letters between doctors don't pull any punches and are just factual. I was reading through it whilst still crouching there with my stomach in a knot, completely transfixed when the postman returned and I nearly jumped out of my skin as a copy of my Will thumped onto the floor next to me. Talk about bad timing! Good job I'm not superstitious. Anyway, I always say it's bad luck to be superstitious!

On the subject of superstition, some years ago, my mother had found a lump in her breast and the doctor, after examining her, said he was arranging for her to see a specialist. My mother tended to worry about things and dwell on the worst-case scenarios. At the time there had been a large sage bush growing in our garden and superstition says that, if the sage bush flourishes, it indicates the woman is the boss in the house. This was a running joke in our family as my mother was very much the boss. As luck would have it, whilst she was worrying about the specialist and whether she had cancer, with my father constantly trying to reassure her, the sage bush suddenly died! As you can imagine, her fears went into overdrive until finally, after listening to her going on and on about the specialist again and asking my father, "What will he be a specialist in?" my father, in frustration said, 'I'll tell you what he's a specialist in, bloody sage bushes!" The lump turned out to be harmless.

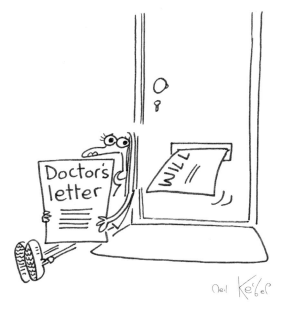

6.   What is the message?

Further down the line, you will have time to reflect on how you got into this situation. I believe that things like cancer don't just 'happen' to us and although you may never be able to pinpoint the exact cause or causes, it's important to reflect on your lifestyle, eating habits, relationships and so on, and gauge how much stress is involved. Look at ways to reduce this stress wherever possible. Stress can be a major factor in ill health and if you've got cancer it can be deadly. It may seem impossible for you to think about changing aspects of your life, such as certain relationships or the way you earn a living, things that cause deep levels of stress, but look at it this way: weigh up each situation and decide whether it's really worth dying for.

In my case, I seemed like the last person in the world who would get cancer. There was no history of cancer in my family, I had a very positive attitude, and I was extremely fit and very disciplined about my eating habits. I've always loved green vegetables even as a child and my three favourite foods are spinach, asparagus and globe artichokes (how about that for luck!) Personally I was in a good, long-term relationship with Alan. Financially, we weren't rich but we certainly had enough to pay for everything we needed without much struggle. Professionally, I was at the top of my game at my practice in Harley Street and running workshops, retreats and training for Chief Executives. I was a very successful professional speaker. What could possibly be wrong with all that?

Reflecting back on things it became clear that my positive attitude was also very driven and being in overdrive was my only gear. Yes, I was very fit which has saved my life on more than one occasion. I had an excellent diet, but I would claim that "I would rather eat nothing than eat rubbish" which resulted in my often doing just that – eating nothing - whilst on my travels running Chief Executive Workshops and retreats. I spent endless hours driving on motorways to the next job.

Arriving home exhausted, I'd often have a glass of wine to wind down and although I wasn't a big drinker, I drank often. So in real terms, although I believed there was method in my madness, in fact there was madness in my method. As someone who has always been self-employed I've found it very difficult to turn down work, there is always the irrational fear of not getting enough of it, so I nearly worked myself to death. I literally got sick to death of being away from home all the time.

I no longer did any painting or drawing, which had been long-term passions. I also stopped other creative things I loved doing, such as sewing, designing, and other crafts. I no longer had the lifestyle to look after Great Danes, dogs which had been a part of my life for over two decades, and I didn't get to go out dancing.

Health-wise there was another factor, which almost certainly didn't help. I'd had an early menopause at the age of forty-six and to my regret, I allowed myself to be persuaded to have synthetic HRT (Synthetic Hormone Replacement Therapy uses chemically altered hormones, rather than 'Bio Identical' hormones which are designed to be 'identical' to our own natural hormones). I know there's controversy over whether HRT causes breast cancer but all I can say is, no one wanted to discuss it once I had breast cancer. My common sense suggests that if there are no possible links between synthetic HRT and breast cancer, why is a history of breast cancer or genetic high risk considered relevant when discussing HRT? I've since discovered that HRT may not cause cancer, but can drive it.

7.   What are you prepared to do to get well?

You have to address every area that isn't conducive to your wellbeing. Take your time to go over every aspect of your life and check whether it feels like joy or stress. Are you constantly sacrificing your own needs to serve others? We all do this to an extent but when it becomes a way of life it becomes life negating. This is what I changed. I became selfish and put my own needs first. It was a matter of life and death. Work-wise, never mind about going the extra mile, in those days, I was ready to go the extra hundred miles. This I had to change. Now, I still go the extra mile, but not the extra hundred.

I also gave up the travelling completely in the short term, and have cut right back on it in the longer term. I may earn less money but what the heck? I spent everything I'd earned on cancer treatments. Therefore I spent more time in my clinic, which is like a home-from-home for me so I continued working there throughout my treatments. I did of course cut out the alcohol. I've become very protective of my time and only turn out for things I really need or want to be at. I made time for friends and other nurturing relationships and got back to art. I still enjoy running and now I tend to organise my time around it rather than trying to find the time to fit it in. I even took up Jive Dancing, it's an amazing de-stresser and a perfect way to get up close and personal with others without the risk of catching anything nasty! I take more time to plan meals and make sure I have plenty of quality food to hand at home. I plan ahead for food to take with me when I'm out and about and I don't allow myself to skip meals. I eliminate anything or any situation that has been the source of unnecessary stress.

8. What are you prepared to do to STAY well?

This is where you have to look at all of the above and consider what you will continue with as part of your normal lifestyle, and what is just a means to an end. I know that some things will be mentally associated with having cancer (I'm no longer fond of Quinoa) but it's important to develop an attitude of healthfulness. (See chapter 5: I don't feel very positive, does that mean I won't make it?). So, for instance, a healthier diet may become a way of life, as could making quality time for friends.

9. What do I want my life to look like from here?

This is the sort of question that needs answering when you're well on the road to recovery and you have more time to reflect. Having had cancer once, it's possible that we're more susceptible. That certainly doesn't mean to me that we should live in constant fear of getting cancer again, however, I view it as a bit like being diabetic in the sense that it's wise to take care of yourself in a healthy and respectful way. As I realise that I may be susceptible, there are some things I'll never do again, such as taking synthetic HRT or using any products containing parabens (oestrogen-mimicking chemicals which have been found in breast cancers and it's unknown for sure how they get there) and other chemicals. I won't allow myself to endure prolonged periods of stress if it can possibly be avoided.

Other things, I'll do only in moderation, such as drinking alcohol, and there are things that I won't be concerned with anymore such as keeping to a very strict diet, which I did in the beginning. Now I just have a healthy eating routine and prioritise buying quality food over other outgoings. It's an appalling insight into our society, that when the credit crunch hit, the first thing people cut back on was the quality of their food.

10. How much will I allow cancer to remain a part of my life?

As you can imagine, or maybe like me you've found out the hard way, you will never be the same after you've had cancer. But there is this bigger question to answer: Do I move on and put the experience behind me or shall I put it to use? Only you can answer this, and it is a very personal thing. Most people, quite understandably, just want to get as far away from it as possible as soon as they can. Because of the nature of my story and my profession I felt that I had to do something with it that would be of service to others. It wasn't completely altruistic, it was the only way that I could make sense of my own experience. Part of me definitely wanted to just get away from it as soon as possible and I thought I'd at least want a bit of breathing space. However, from the beginning, I was willing to talk with others who'd been diagnosed, about the decisions I'd made and to pass on relevant contact details.

As time went on, it naturally followed that many people asked if I'd written anything they could look at, and so this book came into being. It's basically the book I was looking for when I was first diagnosed. I'm not suggesting that everyone should write a book but I know of a lot of people who are willing to be contacted by other cancer patients for support and information. I had contact with a lovely lady who'd been through the same treatment as I had, and had been clear for three and a half years by the time I was diagnosed. She seemed to be a reserved lady who kept herself to herself, but she was kind enough to give me her number. She was a great source of support to me, especially as there is very little official support for those of us who choose an unconventional route. It was a great boost to me to know that she too had experienced good days and bad days just as I was going through, and her physical symptoms had been similar to mine.

Whatever treatment you choose, it's very empowering to have someone to speak to who understands, because they've been there. So you'll find your own answers as to how much cancer remains a part of your life.

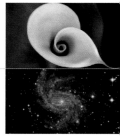
calla lily

spiral galaxy

What do I need to know before I get to the hospital?

Ten actions to take if you've been diagnosed

It's very important to have conversations with your doctors rather than to sit there, like a rabbit in the headlights, waiting to hear your sentence - I mean, treatment programme. I know that at first, we just want them to sort it out and take it all away. We want them to have the answers so we can feel safe again in the hands of beings greater than ourselves with a mysterious knowledge that only they can access. This is a fantasy and, whilst there's nothing wrong with the odd fantasy, being faced with a potentially life threatening situation is not the time to indulge. It's also unfair on the medics who have to live up to these impossible expectations. They're not magicians they're scientists who don't profess to have all the answers.

I would like to make it clear here that, whatever my conversations with doctors, I was in little doubt that they genuinely had my best interests at heart and were doing all they could within their experience, to enable me to survive cancer.

1. Don't be rushed.

Take your time. By this, I don't mean you to leave it indefinitely. I'm merely talking about a couple of weeks, unless you're in an urgent situation and there is no time to spare. This is probably the single most important decision I made. I know that in the first panic of finding out we have cancer we feel we must rush through and get treatment as soon as possible, and get away from the nightmare. I personally felt like there was an invisible hand in my back, pushing me through doors at a rate of knots before I'd had a chance to get my own head around it. When diagnosed, we're all in a serious situation, but few are in an urgent situation. I reasoned that if cancer can take several years to develop, a couple of weeks, one way or the other in order to make sure of the facts, is neither here nor there.

2. Make sure you keep a record of all meetings and consultations.

Keeping track of everything can prove invaluable not just because you can go over information again and think things through, but also because if you see more than one practitioner or consultant it's extremely helpful to have your history to hand with all the medical and additional information. To keep me focussed, I took a companion and a note pad, which was a Christmas gift from a friend, and which I called my 'cancer book'.

It's important to write the date, the name of the hospital or clinic you're visiting, and any consultants' names at the top of the page so that you have a clear record of all the information and treatment you are receiving.

3.   Write down every question.

Write down every question you have and keep your book with you so you can write more questions down as you think of them. Don't make the mistake of thinking you'll do it later as you probably won't remember and there's nothing worse than leaving after a long awaited consultation, only to kick yourself for forgetting to ask something important. Before my appointments, I wrote down every question I could possibly think of. I wrote them down as they came to me through research on the internet, through hearing about other people's experience, thoughts I had in the middle of the night, or anytime anywhere. I just kept my book as my constant companion to make sure I didn't miss anything. I also tended to stick to surgery questions for the surgeon, diet questions for the dietician, and so on. If you don't do this, you risk misinformation.

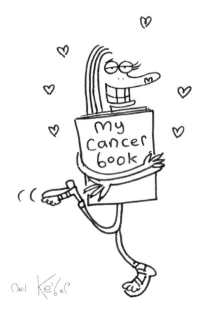

4.   Make sure that you record the answers.

It's a scientific fact that when we're stressed or in shock, we're much less able to function mentally in a calm and reasonable way, because we're in full 'fight or flight' mode. It's all too easy to ask the questions then forget to write down the responses, especially when you're hearing things for the first time, and you're scared witless! During my consultations, I wrote down the answers to my questions, word for word. If you prefer, you can get your companion to do this for you.

5.   Write down more questions during the consultation.

Other questions may arise during the consultation. Sometimes you simply won't know enough to ask the right questions to begin with. I was so keen to get on with the first surgery, a lymph node biopsy (to see if the cancer had spread to the lymph) that I didn't ask enough about it and didn't know enough to ask whether I could get lymphoedema (swelling due to accumulation of lymphatic fluid which can no longer drain away) from the biopsy. I also didn't realise I would be dosed up with morphine (which I have a bad reaction to) during the anaesthetic. I didn't know to ask and so I wasn't told and had to suffer the consequences. (12 hours of severe vomiting after surgery, combined with a migraine headache and slight underarm swelling with accompanying discomfort a couple of times a year due to lymphatic build up).

Consultants are usually very open to giving as much information as possible but they are not mind readers. You need to tell them if there's anything specific you need to go over.

6.   If you don't understand something, ask them to clarify.

No matter how confused or muddled you may feel, keep asking until you have some clarity in your own mind. YOU are ultimately responsible for what happens to YOU. I had an intense discussion about a mastectomy which was a change from the surgeons' original recommendation which was a lumpectomy (removal of lump.) Confused and upset, I mentioned that I was being told something different at every meeting I had. The nurse replied that, "cancer treatment is not an exact science". Well, you don't say! Nevertheless, I felt I was expected to take some pretty big risks for something they didn't seem too sure about.

Don't be concerned about asking too many questions, even if your consultant or doctor becomes irritated. Remember that although it may all be in a day's work for them, you are hearing it for the first time and have to make some major life decisions based on their information. It's also difficult to keep a clear mind through the emotion of a cancer diagnosis. For instance, I found I was automatically booked in for chemotherapy. This is mainly the case with cancer treatment and I understand that it works this way because most people don't question anything, they just assume that it's the right way and for the best. Personally I felt like I was just being 'processed' like everyone else and was no longer an individual. Most people accept treatment in the belief that it's the only way. It was assumed that I would just allow it all to happen as if I was part of a computerised process, where my details had been entered and the treatment programme spat out and I was duly expected to sleepwalk through the whole thing. If you wish to be treated as an individual you must individuate yourself.

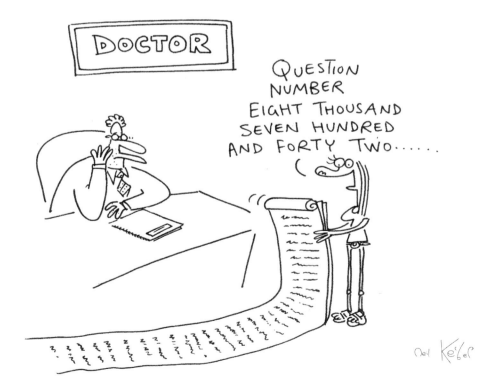

7.   Don't assume that what you are told is the only way or the best way for you.

I know it seems easier to have the attitude, "I don't want to know anything just let them get on with it," but you have to remember that you and you alone have to live with the results and the potential impact on your life. Remember, it's not their life, it's yours!

This reminds me of how I decided against chemotherapy. I was automatically booked in for it and when I went to the oncologist for assessment, I was told the resident oncologist was away so I saw a replacement. The young man examined me and declared that apart from having cancer, I was extremely healthy. He told me about the recommended treatment (AC-accelerated Taxolchemotherapy, in two parts) and that it would be accelerated in the second half (this means repeated every two weeks instead of every three) as recommended by my consultant. I asked the oncologist how my treatment would benefit me, how would it increase my chances of survival. He replied that it would only increase it by up to 7%, compared with the survival chances of not having chemotherapy at all.

At this point the breast cancer nurse assured me that her relative had just had a bi-lateral mastectomy (both breasts removed) with chemotherapy and radiotherapy and she was, "absolutely fine!" I chose not to respond to this statement. She seemed agitated that I was asking so many plain questions to which the oncologist responded honestly and directly. This was understandable up to a point, his answers were quite grim and she was doing her level best to help me to feel more confident and positive.

The oncologist also told me that they don't really have the figures to give accurate answers which surprised me, considering that chemotherapy has, to my knowledge, been used for about fifty years! I then asked how they had decided on my treatment programme, and he told me it was a computer programme (and not a very up to date one at that). Then I asked him what details were fed into the programme and he told me it was my age, whether I was pre or post-menopausal, and the size and grade of my tumour. I asked him why chemotherapy was recommended for me, given the only slightly better chance of survival and the appalling risks associated with the 'therapy'. He answered that at that particular time they were trailling the effectiveness of using chemotherapy before surgery rather than after it, in order to shrink the tumour and necessitate less extensive surgery. Apparently, they were hoping to find out whether this increased overall survival levels. In fact, I've since found out that shrinking a tumour with chemotherapy prior to surgery has no impact on survival levels. I need to mention here that in medical terms, 'survival' is taken to mean still being alive five years after diagnosis. It doesn't mean, as one would like to think, that survival means you're cured and will live happily ever after.

It seemed I was supposed to accept what I considered to be unreasonable risks to my health simply to keep more of my breast, a purely cosmetic issue, as I saw it. These risks included a depleted immune system, possible tissue damage from chemotherapy leaking out of veins, memory and concentration impairment, damage to heart muscle, serious blood disorders such as leukaemia and many other shorter term horrors such as tiredness, muscle aches, eye irritation and hair loss. I told the oncologist that although I didn't relish losing most of or my entire breast, I was 50 years old and not a 19 year old page three girl, so to risk serious and permanent health damage, or even death in the hope of ending up with a better pair of jugs was hardly my priority.

He agreed that I should think about it very carefully. I then asked the 'six million dollar question'. "If you were in my situation" I said, "would you accept chemotherapy? "No." was his reply. At this point the nurse pointed out that I was obviously very intelligent, and she stopped trying to sugarcoat the story. Don't get me wrong here, she was a wonderful nurse and very professional and was doing her best to help me come to terms with a grim situation. I'm just a lousy patient who wouldn't play ball. I walked out of there hugely relieved having made the decision that I was in no way going to submit to chemotherapy, and no-one had given me what I would consider a reasonable or rational explanation as to why I should. The numbers simply didn't add up and I had no interest in being a part of that 'trial'.

8. Check your paperwork.

No matter how scary it seems, check it over and over again to make absolutely sure you know what's happening and why. I remember going over a surgeon's letter describing the lumpectomy (removal of the cancerous lump or tumour) and, even after my careful notes and questioning and copies of their letters, I noticed for the first time that they planned a latissimusdorsi reconstruction (taking a piece of tissue from under my shoulder blade to help reconstruct the breast) This would have been a bigger surgery than I had thought, with other implications such as healing time, more reconstructive surgery and extra scarring on my back. How could I have missed this?

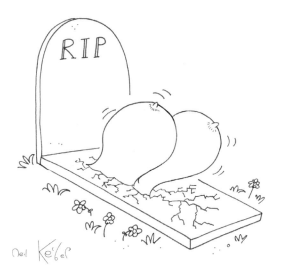

9. After every appointment, take time, check what you think has happened, and compare notes with your companion.

When we have to take in a huge amount of information, quickly and in an emotionally stressful situation, it really helps to allow time for the information to sink in. This can be enhanced by distracting yourself with a book or TV or a different kind of conversation before you go back to the subject in hand with some fresh energy.

I found this process helped me round out my thinking and keep things in perspective. It's important to mention here that you should choose a companion who can be objective and who supports you in whatever decisions you choose to make. I remember one lady who'd had a mastectomy (removal of her breast) and had chosen to do the rest of her treatment alternatively as she didn't want chemotherapy or radiotherapy. She was put in touch with me so we could support each other. She told me, on our first meeting that some of her family were refusing to speak to her because she wouldn't have conventional treatment. Really! She needed that about as much as she needed another hole in her backside!

Before you have surgery, if you're not sure of anything, don't be afraid to have another talk with your consultant to clarify exactly what's going to happen. This is ultimately your responsibility. It's a bit late to find afterwards that you've had surgery you weren't expecting. They can't put things back inside or sew them back on so read your paperwork and make sure that you understand what it all means.

When I had a lymph node biopsy (a small number of lymph nodes surgically removed from my underarm to check for spread of cancer), a diagnostic procedure which was my only surgery, they removed three lymph nodes and found one contained a single cell, one contained a micro metastasis (a small cluster of cancer cells) and the third contained nothing. When they told me the results I was assured that it would be extremely unlikely that there would be anything in the other lymph nodes but they would like to remove them "just for safety". I was unconvinced and explained that as far as I understood it, if I got cancer again, it would probably be in the same place, so my lymph nodes, which are part of my immune system, were pretty important. Therefore I was loath to have my immune system compromised where I needed it the most. There was also the very real risk of lymphodoema (swelling of the arm due to build-up of lymphatic fluid which is uncomfortable, unsightly and permanent). I told him I wasn't sure and needed to think about it. Anyway, the letter sent to my GP stated that:

"…and certainly, examining her again today she is suitable for breast conservation with all the small risks associated with that. …In regard to her axilla we do not yet know the full implications of micro metastases in the sentinel node setting and that completion axillary dissection may be an option for her (removal of the lymph nodes from my underarm). She is in agreement with this and is happy to undertake the procedure at the same time."

There is now new research which suggests that lymph node removal does not extend life.

The surgery was booked in and I got in touch with the surgeon's secretary to say that I hadn't agreed to it. She arranged another meeting with the surgeons, four days prior to the planned surgery. In the meantime, I'd started the metabolic therapy, which meant an alkaline diet. (See chapter 4) Within three weeks the tumour changed from an impenetrable, hard, calcified lump to a soft, jelly like mass. I didn't mention my diet at the meeting and, when they examined me they completely changed their recommendation from a lumpectomy to a mastectomy! It was clear that one surgeon wasn't entirely in agreement but the other was more senior, so he conceded. The senior surgeon was understandably frustrated with me by now, finally saying "Oh why don't you just have a mastectomy and get it over with". And who could blame him? He was giving me the best advice he could, based on his training, skills and experience, and here was I dithering around and risking my life, as more and more time was passing.

The breast cancer nurse then asked me, "Now then Jessica, what is it that bothers you about a mastectomy?" I angrily replied. "The same thing that would bother you about it I expect!" Then she said. "You're no different from anyone else, everyone resists it at first but they all come to terms with it." I chose not to respond. I was then asked if there was any way I'd consider having chemotherapy, and the nurse added that a lot of people tolerate it well. Still angry, I said. "Well bully for them!" I told the remaining surgeon that I needed to think about the surgery and would let him know.

I needed to check whether the change to the tumour was a sign that the metabolic therapy was working. I didn't want to risk having an unnecessary mastectomy. I was still in a state of shock when the second surgeon said. "Well, it's good that we have these extra meetings because sometimes we do need to make slight adjustments." I said. "Slight adjustments? One's with a tit and one's without a tit, that's a bit more than a slight adjustment!" The poor man looked horrified and said I should phone him to discuss it further. He was a very compassionate and patient person. (He's now a consultant at another hospital and I know his patients are lucky to have such a kind surgeon. I'm sure he will have a very positive impact on his patients). The lymph node issue was still unresolved.

10. Get a second, third or fourth opinion.

After the last meeting I called Dr Andre and asked if the softening of the tumour was expected now that I was on the metabolic diet. He confirmed that this was so, but he encouraged me to get a second opinion from a medic who hadn't examined me before. He advised me to go to a new hospital and see a new consultant. My GP got me an appointment and in the meantime I spoke with another patient of Dr Andre's, who reversed her breast cancer using the same method as myself and, at the time, had been clear for about three and a half years. She told me that exactly the same thing had happened to her tumour when she started the metabolic therapy and that it meant the treatment was working.

Then I called Phillip Day, from whom I'd got a lot of relevant, up to date information, and he confirmed that he'd heard the same thing many times from patients starting metabolic therapy. I felt relieved and a lot more confident after these conversations.

When I finally got to the new consultant, it was clear from the outset that he was extremely hostile. He began by attacking me verbally for daring to first go elsewhere when his was a far better hospital. He also said that he didn't know what I was doing there anyway as I didn't want conventional treatment. He assured me that nine other women he knew had taken a combined or alternative route and they were all dead! (He didn't mention how many taking the conventional route had also died in the same period of time). He examined me and said that chemotherapy and a mastectomy was the only way as well as having all my lymph nodes removed. I was lymph positive and therefore had an even lower chance of survival. He then informed me that I'd probably already left it too late as every three months that passed after diagnosis had greatly reduced my chances of survival and I was already four months down the line. I have to confess that I felt so angry at the time over his bullying and arrogant attitude I remember thinking that, at that moment, *he* was a lot closer to death than I was!

But I said nothing as I was there for the scan. During the scan I asked the radiologist if he could tell whether the tumour was active or inactive and he agreed to have a look. He showed me the extent of the tumour and pointed out that it was lying flat against the tissues. Then he looked up at me and smiled, and told me it meant the tumour wasn't active and that it was a good sign that my treatment was working.

There was no mention of his comments when I went back in to see the consultant whose verdict was that "it's still the same size, so my treatment is a waste of time."

Of course, I had no intention of remaining his patient. The idea of leaving my unconscious body in the hands of that antagonistic bully armed with a scalpel didn't require much deliberation. I eventually realised that I should try to see the consultant who was treating the woman using the same treatment I was, who had agreed to let me contact her. Surely her consultant had some experience of monitoring someone who recovered using the same treatment. My poor GP once again wrote for a referral and I was thrilled when I later got an appointment.

When I met this man for our first consultation, I was faced with kindness personified. He quietly asked me to tell him the story of how I got to him. He examined me thoroughly (this was a first) asked questions and asked for my notes, (which I'd brought with me) in order that he could have them copied. At the end of the consultation he told me that, having run the biggest lymph node trial in existence, (more than 1,000 surgeries) and never finding anything more in patients like myself, he agreed that I should not have any more lymph nodes removed as, in his opinion, it was not worth the risk. He added, "However, we shall remember that the enemy has visited." He told me that he didn't know if I would survive or succumb, that only time would tell, but, at that time I was not in an urgent situation. Then he ordered a full spectrum of blood tests (the only consultant who did so) and said he would see me again two months later for more blood tests and an ultrasound scan which I'd requested. When we left the clinic I had no doubt that I'd found the right consultant for me.

Although he didn't promote alternative treatments and said what I was doing was, in his opinion, "unscientific" he would nevertheless monitor me with the clear understanding that, should I notice any changes or find that my treatment wasn't working, I should let him know immediately to ensure I didn't miss an opportunity for surgery and conventional treatment. I agreed to his terms.

He remains my consultant to this day.

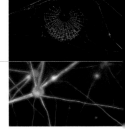

CHAPTER 3

I have an appointment at the hospital: What do I ask?

Ten Questions to ask the Doctors

A cancer diagnosis can leave you speechless, but don't stay that way. You are facing a very serious situation with some very serious decisions to make. You can of course, hand everything over to your consultants and leave them to make all your decisions for you. You can tell them that you don't want to know the details, you just want them to get on with it and get it over with. And who could blame you? I certainly wouldn't. The thing is though, there is no getting away from it and unless you go forward with your eyes open, you could find yourself facing a situation you didn't expect. Ultimately, it's your body and your life, and you alone will have to deal with the outcomes of decisions made, whether you make them yourself or leave them to others.

It seems to me that cancer is such a common disease that it's almost impossible to be treated as an individual, especially if you don't actively take part in your own treatment programme. How can it be otherwise when a limited system has to deal with over 40,000 new breast cancer cases alone every year?

For your own sake, ask the questions which will enable you to make the best decisions for yourself. Then you will gain the greatest understanding of your own situation, and your best chance of recovery.

Before you begin, from a medical point of view, the first thing is to choose the hospital and consultant. Take your time with this. It amazes me how most of us are willing to put our life in the hands of someone we happened to have allocated to us, based on being the first consultant available at the nearest hospital. Would you take your car to a garage based purely on the fact that it was the nearest? Would you buy a computer after seeing it in a shop window without any further research? Think about it.

I also want to stress here that if your consultant is unhappy about answering your questions or treats you less than respectfully, then change him or her. It's unlikely you will need to do this as, in my experience, with one exception, I found the medical staff to be extremely helpful, patient and understanding, always willing to assist me in any way they could. However, if you have to, keep looking until you find someone who's experienced and sympathetic as well as respectful.

1.   What *exactly* is my diagnosis?

Being diagnosed with cancer isn't enough in itself. It's important to know what kind of cancer it is and what, in the doctors' experience is the usual course of treatment, and the expected outcome. This will give you a basic idea of what the normal medical thinking and beliefs are regarding your diagnosis. Surprisingly, much medical treatment is based on belief rather than fact. For instance, it was a belief that chemotherapy, surgery and radiotherapy were the only course of action available to me and to convince me of this I was told, "You can't cut corners with this thing." There was no other way. But that was just his experience.

I will mention more than once in this book that in my opinion, medical research can be flawed. Very little data is taken into account. For instance, thousands of breast cancer cases are treated according to trials which only take into account a person's age, whether they are pre or post-menopausal and the size and stage of their tumour. I was told, for instance that chemotherapy could improve my chances of survival by up to 7%. No account was being taken of the varying lifestyles, economic and social status, dietary habits, body type and characteristics of the individuals involved, and no note was made of those who died during the course of their treatment.

2.   How did I get cancer?

It seems to me that the only truthful answer to this is, "I don't know". When I asked this question I was told it was, 'A roll of the dice'. Well, that didn't really cut it for me. It was said during my first consultation with a consultant surgeon and, until this point, he'd been quoting science at me and recommending some pretty severe treatment which would go on for at least a year. I began to lose confidence, as I wondered how I could be expected to bet my life on treatment prescribed in the *belief* that the disease I had was caused simply by chance! Not a very scientific explanation. The consultant wasn't deliberately being vague, his answer was simply based on his belief.

His belief may be based on his experience, which is understandable, but, until I was in my twenties, my experience of the sea was that it's cold and brown (and I wouldn't have been blamed for having that belief) until I went abroad and found out otherwise!

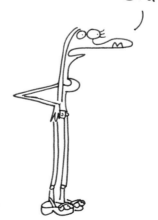

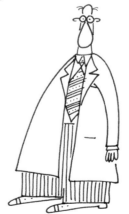

3. What are the side effects of the chemotherapy?

You will usually be given a printed handout explaining the possible effects of the particular chemotherapy agent recommended for you. It is important that you look into this very carefully so that you can weigh up the level of risk you're prepared to take. In many cases, chemotherapy will not improve your chances of survival by much and you will need to decide if you would stand a better chance without it.

Remember: in medical terms, 'survival' simply means still being alive five years after diagnosis. It's important to note here that as far as research is concerned, it would be very difficult to get a true number because you would have to take say, one hundred cancer patients and have fifty of them have chemotherapy and the other fifty not, in order to see some kind of result. Even then, many other factors would have to be taken into account, such as type of cancer, age and health of the patient, mental attitude, diet and so on. So the numbers can only be based on those who have chemotherapy.

So what are the longer term side effects of chemotherapy? This is a very important question, as you can be left with long-term health issues. In my case, I was leaving myself open to a small but none the less possible risk of leukaemia associated with Taxol chemotherapy. Remember also that toxic agents like chemotherapy have to be metabolised by the body in order to eliminate them and this means that they have to be processed by either your liver or kidneys or both, depending on the type of chemotherapy used. This can cause permanent damage to those organs. Chemotherapy, in most cases, is designed to bring you to the point of death in order to destroy as much of the cancer as possible. This, I discovered was why the fitter a person is the more will be thrown at them in the belief they can tolerate more without dying, therefore giving them a better chance by destroying more of the cancer.

This makes sense on one level if one believes there is no other way. But check out your own situation. From my perspective at the time I felt it presented an unacceptable risk to my health. I knew that there was no doubt that chemotherapy agents can and do kill some cancer cells, but I calculated that in my case, the risks were too high at the time.

4. Assuming my treatment is successful, will I have a normal life expectancy? What are the percentages?

This is a difficult one, as the answer may vary from one consultant to the next but it's still worth asking so that you can gauge whether it's the right way for you or, after investigation, whether you feel you can improve on their figures by choosing different or complementary treatments.

Always ask what the percentage chance of success is in the case of your chemotherapy. Everyone I've spoken to expects the answer to this to be from 40% - 90% (given the severity of the side effects) and are horrified to find that at best, it's only up to 7%! (I'm referring to breast cancer here) This can vary with different cancers. Testicular cancer for example can have up to a 90% success rate with chemotherapy.

5. How many people die from the effects of chemotherapy?

This is an interesting one as, to my knowledge, chemotherapy is never recorded as a cause of death. Death of cancer patients is always attributed to cancer.

6.   What's usually the long term plan?

After much discussion with a breast cancer consultant, I asked this question and was a little dismayed by the response, given the amount of treatment I was expected to subject myself to, especially as this same consultant had told me at the beginning that, "You can't cut corners with a thing like this". In answer to my question, I was told that there would be no blood tests (I found out that private patients at the same hospital with the same consultant did receive blood tests) I would only have regular mammograms to check if the cancer returned. (I'm unconvinced about the safety of mammograms as they can deliver up to 1,000 times the dose of radiation one would get from a normal chest X-Ray) I did not feel greatly encouraged by this.

7.   How effective would you expect radiation to be in cases such as mine?

Again, this has to be carefully weighed up. Radiation can kill some cancer cells but will also cause damage to healthy tissue. However, these days it has been greatly refined for accuracy and in breast cancer it can be aimed tangentially, so as to avoid penetration of deeper tissues not affected by cancer. On the other hand, when first diagnosed, I was advised to have radiotherapy as part of my treatment but when I changed to the metabolic diet, the tumour, which had been hard and calcified, broke down to a jelly like mass within three weeks and I was then advised that a mastectomy would be the safest option for me given that there was now a high risk there would be cancer cells in the 'margin' (the centimetre of healthy tissue taken around the tumour) I was now told that the other benefit of a mastectomy would mean that I'd no longer need radiotherapy. It was explained that this would be a big plus, as radiotherapy could cause heart damage due to the fact my heart is enlarged

after years of running, and in addition, the radiation would almost guarantee lymphoedema (a build-up of lymphatic fluid which is painful, compromises the immune system and makes one susceptible to infection should that area be scratched or damaged in some way) in that arm.

So, check the risks and weigh them up against the benefits before you decide if it's the best choice for you.

The biggest problem I had with the idea of radiotherapy was that my father had, for many years been a radiographer in a nuclear power station, so I learned from an early age of the dangers of radiation, the main one being that Radiation causes Cancer! This made it almost impossible for me to see exposure to radiation as a 'therapy'. There are of course, many types of radiation and many different methods of using it, however my experience and background knowledge of the subject would no doubt, have had a negative effect on the outcome of my treatment. So, making these decisions is such a personal thing.

8.   How long have you treated cancer patients?

I set a lot of store on the amount of actual experience a healthcare practitioner may have (whether it's conventional or otherwise) bearing in mind that their experience may be limited to a specialised area. It is less important to me how qualified a person may be, because when it comes down to brass tacks, I prefer to have the opinion of someone who's performed that surgery many times before or who's dealt with many cases similar to my own. I certainly feel more confident in experienced hands and in having questions answered by the voice of experience. It amazes me that we ask more questions about a car or a new computer before we buy it and wouldn't put either in the hands of another for repair without checking they have the knowledge and experience to deal with them yet, when it comes to our health and even our lives, we accept anyone and anything without question! What's that all about?

Ask your consultant about his/her experience, and what are the commonalities, if any in patients who recover. This is where experience really comes into its own, although we have to bear in mind that not only can different cancers behave very differently but the same cancers can also behave very differently in individual cases. Nevertheless, an experienced consultant/healthcare practitioner would notice over the years, certain characteristics in disease, treatment and nature of patients which are more common in those who recover. It's worth taking note of, in case there's anything you can add which could enhance your own situation.

9. What is your opinion of diet and nutrition?

As you may have already read, I'm big on nutrition as a major part of any recovery programme and if you feel the same way, you need to know if you're 'singing from the same hymn sheet' as your consultant or health care practitioner. Now, your consultant may know little about diet and nutrition but usually they will have an open mind and be happy that you are including anything that may help you, as long as it will do you no harm. On the other hand, if they are dismissive or even disrespectful with regard to diet and nutrition, or appear to have a closed mind, then you might want to consider whether you are with the right person.

10. Would you subject yourself to this treatment if you had cancer or were in a similar situation to myself?

This is a big one but, again, in other areas of life, we have no problem asking a professional what they would do in a similar situation, say, with regard to a car or a computer, but it rarely occurs to us to ask such a question with regard to our health. I asked my heating engineer if he would bother with insurance two years after a boiler like mine had been installed and he replied that I didn't need it as those boilers are built to last and a regular service would be sufficient. He said he wouldn't bother if it were his.

So, ask your consultant. As you may have already read, when I asked an oncologist if he would have chemotherapy in the same situation as myself he replied that he wouldn't!

I also asked, what would happen if I did nothing at all, and was told that, if it spread to my brain, it would kill me very quickly whereas if it spread to a rib, it could be there for several years before becoming terminal. Apparently, there was no real way of knowing. However, I've included this question as, should I find myself in a situation which is deemed terminal by conventional standards, I would have to evaluate whether any treatment being offered would simply prolong my life by a few miserable weeks or months or whether I could choose another course and keep myself well for as long as possible. It's a very personal choice between length of life vs. quality of life and we can only base it on our own feelings and circumstances at the time.

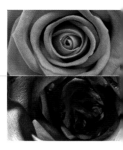

CHAPTER 4

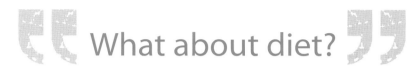

What about diet?

Ten things to eat and why,
Ten things not to eat and why

PLUS: Ten recipes to get you started, and a great store cupboard list.

These days, nobody in their right mind would argue with the fact that diet and nutrition have a profound effect on our state of health and wellbeing. The media constantly bombards us, as research proves beyond a doubt that this is the case. A good healthy diet, which is mainly alkaline, is great if you are well but some of the more specialised diets are helpful if you have cancer.

In my opinion and experience, after mental attitude, diet and nutrition play the biggest part in recovery from most illnesses. Every cell in our bodies is made up from what we eat and drink so it's completely irrational to imagine that what you eat and drink has no effect on your state of health and general wellbeing. Look at it this way; if you have diabetes, you must address your diet, if you have a heart condition, you will be given dietary advice but if you have cancer, or most other diseases for that matter, no such thing happens. How can diet be recognised as having an impact on some diseases and not others? I asked at one cancer hospital if they gave nutritional advice, if they had a nutritionist and if they were affiliated to any nutritional organisation. I was told by the doctor and nurse that they were not trained or qualified in that area, they didn't know anything about it and were not affiliated to any relevant organisation which could offer that advice. The nurse then immediately assured me that it didn't matter, as it made no difference what you ate or drank! (She'd just told me she knew nothing about it and wasn't qualified to give advice).

What follows is basic information, with brief explanations to get you started.

NB: I STRONGLY RECOMMEND THAT YOU FOLLOW THE ADVICE OF A QUALIFIED NUTRITIONIST IN ORDER TO HAVE A PLAN ADAPTED TO YOUR NEEDS AND REQUIREMENTS AND THE TYPE OF CANCER YOU ARE DEALING WITH.

The idea of a specialist cancer diet is to support the immune system and at the same time create a hostile environment to the cancer within the body. If you are having conventional treatment, your diet can increase the efficacy of your treatments whilst reducing the side effects. My nutritional plan was based on the Gerson Therapy, a tried and tested regime of long standing. Many anti-cancer diets are based on this regime. The World Cancer Research Fund has some excellent information on recommended diets for cancer. Also check out Cancer Active, and Breast Cancer Haven. (see Resources: p111)

I want to make it clear that I'm not suggesting all these products cause cancer, only that it's very important to be aware of the effect some of these products can have in a cancer environment. One thing I will say, is that if you make the decision to use diet as part of your treatment, then take full responsibility and stick to it wholeheartedly. Don't mess around with it, there are no half measures. We're not children, we're adults dealing with a life and death situation!

Ten things not to eat and why

1. sugar

Cancer cells are anaerobic and glucose-receptive which basically means that cancer cells are dependent on sugar rather than oxygen for growth. In other words, if you want to feed cancer cells then sugar in its various forms is the ideal! If you experience sugar cravings whilst on the diet, remembering why you are on your diet will make it easy to resist.

I just put up with the cravings and stuck to the diet. After all, it wasn't a case of trying to resist in order not to put on a few pounds, I just asked myself whether I wanted to feed the cancer cells. Remember to check with your nutritionist as some grains and root vegetables can also be high in sugar. (By the way, one of my occasional indulgences these days is a few squares of raw chocolate which is available at most good health food shops).

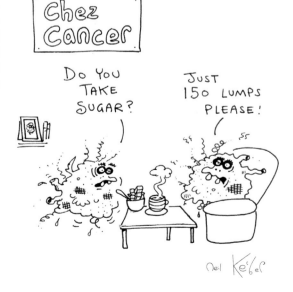

2. alcohol

Far from needing alcohol, it is actually toxic to the body and is a highly refined form of sugar so if you want to suppress your immune system and feed the cancer cells, consuming alcohol is a good way to start. Again, consuming a small amount of alcohol may be fine combined with a healthy diet but we're not just talking about healthy diets here, we're talking about a specialised and targeted anti cancer regime. I remember someone trying to persuade me that a small glass of wine wouldn't hurt, and under ordinary circumstances this was probably true but in my case it could have completely disrupted the sugar-free environment I'd created over nearly a year.

In the body, alcohol may cause DNA damage, which in turn can cause cancer.

3. tea

We're talking about black tea here (builders tea), as this can have an acidic effect on the body. Green tea and white tea and herbal teas are fine, especially if they are organic. Black tea isn't bad as such but you are dealing with a low acid, high alkaline specialist diet. I'm actually a big fan of tea and these days, I do enjoy the odd cup of black tea with no milk or sugar. I buy a good quality organic brand from the supermarket. Black tea is actually very rich in anti-oxidants and also works as an antibiotic which is why without it, we probably wouldn't have even had an industrial revolution, let alone led one. During those times, people were living in the cities in very cramped and unhygienic situations, without sanitation, in order to get the work in mills and factories. Disease would have been rife, were it not due to the fact that British workers drank on average a couple of pints of tea per day which acted as a constant supply of antibiotics. The Brits were not known for their water drinking habits, it was either tea or beer even for children. So, just lay off tea if you have cancer.

4. yeast

This will cause fermentation in the gut, which in turn creates an acidic environment in the body. Cancer cells as well as yeasts love an acidic environment. You will be amazed how many things contain yeast so read packets carefully. If you shop in supermarkets, I can save you the trouble; you will find yeast hidden in almost everything you fancy. In particular, you will need to go to specialist health food shops to buy your yeast-free bread, making sure it is baked with grains allowed on your diet. Also check things such as stock cubes, which will contain yeast. Yeast free stock cubes are available in health food shops, but they're not so easy to find in supermarkets nowadays. Stock cubes are a godsend when you're making all the vegetable and pulse soups, but check you are allowed them on your diet as they do contain salt.

Doctor, I cut out yeast.
Here, I baked you a nice big
loaf of bread
to say thank you!

Neil Kerber

5. coffee

As with tea, except that coffee has even more chemicals (especially if it's decaffeinated) and higher levels of caffeine, especially in the amounts that we drink it. Having said that, there are some schools of thought which recommend a small cup of coffee once per day as part of a cancer recovery programme. It all depends on the nutritionist you choose and the programme which feels right for you. I chose to cut it out for the time being but am looking forward to enjoying the odd cup of good Italian coffee in the future.

6. processed foods

Not only are processed foods generally of poor nutritional value, but the additives cause acidity in the body and depress the immune system. Processed foods mean just that, foods which have gone through a process which alters them from their original state, such as many fast food items. Many processed foods also contain high levels of sugar and/or salt as well as yeast and, even worse, hydrogenated vegetable oils which can suppress your immune system. Do try to keep your food as fresh and as near its natural state as possible.

A good deal of wholesome Asian cuisine works very well with a metabolic diet as it doesn't tend to include a great deal of meat or dairy but does include a high amount of fresh, lightly cooked vegetables as well as delicious, health enhancing spices.

7. old food

If food has been left lying around for too long its nutritional value can be zero. To build new and healthy cells, the body requires fresh wholesome food free from additives and chemicals. Don't hang on to old food in your fridge, keep it stocked with fresh produce. Try to ensure it is fresh when you buy it. I order an organic box of veg weekly and I know its contents are never more than a day or so old when it arrives. We also have a wonderful veg shop in the small town square where I live which sells fresh, organic veg and what they term 'field produce', which is basically fruit and veg grown locally without the use of chemicals, in private gardens, allotments or community gardens so, although it's not 'officially' organic it's certainly as good as, and has often just been picked that morning.

8. dead food

Dead food is the same as old food except that you will find it in shops rather than your fridge. You cannot expect your body to produce healthy cells from nutritionally dead food. In general, this includes all foods and drinks which no longer resemble their original state. They are laden with what are called 'empty calories' which basically means calories with no nutritional content. Apart from anything else, consuming these kinds of foods is a fast way to become fat. When we get hungry, it's the body's signal that it requires nutrition. If we feed it calories without nutrition the calories have to be stored in the form of fat and you know where that goes - on your bum, tum and thighs. You will quickly become hungry again because your body is still crying out for nutrition so you can guess what happens when you feed it yet more empty calories. And so the cycle continues, your body is effectively being starved as your fat stores grow ever larger along with all the problems that entails.

9. fizzy drinks and squashes

These are basically sugar and chemicals. You can work this one out for yourself. These drinks are often recommended to cancer patients who, because of chemotherapy and other treatments have a much-compromised immune system, because there is nothing live contained in them. The thinking behind this is that with such a compromised immune system a microbe from fresh food or drink could prove life threatening so patients are advised to eat and drink only dead substances. Whilst I understand the thinking behind this, my issue is that this was the only nutritional advice I saw of any description.

Whilst waiting for pre surgical assessment at one of the major cancer hospitals accompanied by my friend Marisa we were offered tea, coffee, sandwiches and various other refreshments. We were curious to have a look at the menu, which advised the following; *if you are having chemotherapy, or have leukaemia or other immune deficiencies, do not consume any live food including water. Eat only sweets, chocolates, biscuits and crisps and drink only canned fizzy drinks!* This was the only dietary advice I saw at this hospital and explained the huge vending machines packed full of the stuff.

It's interesting to note that when I did find nutritional information for cancer patients, the diet guide listed such things as pizza with extra cheese, Angel Delight, and ready made chocolate desserts such as Aero, Rolo and Dairy Milk, cake, oven or microwave chips and crisps, (although the guide also had an eight step plan for healthy eating if you have cancer, as recommended by the World Cancer Research Fund, one of my recommended websites by the way). However, underneath the plan, is a picture supplied by the Food Standards Agency, which shows that more than a third of our diet should be bread, pasta and dairy, as well as food and drinks containing sugar!

As I mentioned earlier, some forms of treatment can cause loss of appetite, nausea and weight loss, so that's why fortified products are added to the recipes, but if you remember it's all a patient is eating, the sample recipes were, to say the least, unappealing.

For instance, Cold Peach Pudding , is made by pouring 'Esure Plus' over madeira cake, and adding tinned peaches and double cream. And Coffee Calypso is a combination of a sachet of Vanilla 'Build-Up' a third of a pint of whole milk, 6tsp glucose polymer powder, a scoop of ice cream and 1-2 teaspoons of instant coffee. Now that is alarming.

10. dairy

Dairy means products which come from the cow. It doesn't include eggs, as some people believe just because these are often put with dairy products in supermarkets. Not only do milk and cheese create acidity but cheese is also full of microbes which add to the gut problems and acidity. It's especially not a good idea to ingest dairy products if you have a hormonally driven cancer, such as breast or prostate, as dairy products are full of hormones including growth hormones which all milk has in order for the baby animal to grow. A cow is a big animal so its growth hormones are probably the last thing you would want if you have a tumour. Some nutritionists will advise in some cases that a small amount of goats' cheese is acceptable but again, you will have to make your own call on that.

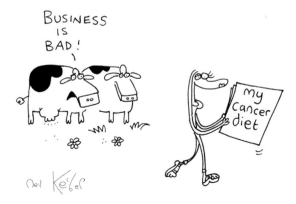

Neil Kerber

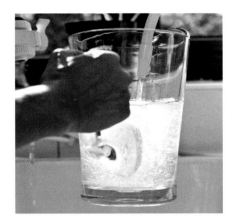

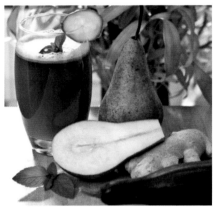

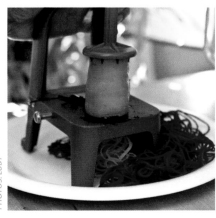

PHOTOS: LUBY

1. water

Never underestimate the value of drinking water, especially purified or bottled water (although bottled water can often be of a poorer quality than some tap water and some of it actually is tap water). I could write a whole chapter on tap water and all the added chemicals and their effects but suffice it to say that I only use Kangen water and have a system installed in my home for drinking, cooking and other household purposes. I have no doubt this is the single most important investment I've made for my continued excellent health. (for more information on Kangen water go to www.jessicarichards.co.uk)

Dehydration can have long term devastating effects on health. Most people do not drink enough water. Fizzy drinks, coffee and tea and so on don't count as fluid intake as far as hydration is concerned. In fact, some drinks actually have a dehydrating effect on the body. The general rule is, one should drink a cup of water for every cup of tea (this doesn't include herbal, green or white teas) and two cups of water for every cup of coffee. This doesn't count as hydration but simply cancels out the dehydrating effects of the tea and coffee. This information is not usually available within the medical environment.

During some forms of chemotherapy, it's very important to drink plenty of fluid as the chemotherapy agent is metabolised through the kidneys and therefore the kidneys need to be flushed out with fluid throughout the treatment. An older lady I knew was advised that this was the case with her chemotherapy treatment and, like most older people she drank very little on a daily basis so when she arrived at the hospital she was told to have a cup of hot chocolate! How about that - a cup of sugary chemicals in milk when plain water would have been ideal.

2. vegetable juice

I mean fresh vegetable juice please, not the canned stuff. There's nothing wrong with that but again, we are dealing with a cancer recovery program here so different rules apply. Green vegetable juice is alkalising, releases and eliminates toxins and provides antioxidants and nutrients directly into your system. I make one, large juice per day. Some anti-cancer regimes recommend several per day or even one per hour, but for me, there has to be more to life than sitting in front of a juicer every waking hour! You'll have to decide what works best for you.

Try to ensure that all your ingredients are fresh and organic. If you can't afford organic or if it's not available, soak your ingredients for about ten minutes in water and cider vinegar to remove residual chemicals. Buy the best juicer you can afford and don't confuse a juicer with a blender. A blender is for blending ingredients whereas a juicer extracts the juice. (You will however find a blender invaluable for making smoothies and soups)

There are many juicing books available with various recipes but for practicalities sake, this is my basic recipe:

1 whole cucumber
piece of fresh ginger to taste
stump of broccoli, cabbage or other piece of greenery.
1 small beetroot
1 small pear

Juice all ingredients raw. Enjoy!

You can also have wheatgrass juice, which is normally drunk only in small 'shot' glasses. It is alkaline, and extremely high in chlorophyll which will encourage the production of red blood cells. You can either grow your own or buy the trays (a heck of a lot easier.)

3. green leafy vegetables

These can literally be a lifesaver. They are alkalizing, and full of chlorophyll as well as other nutrients and enzymes. Chlorophyll acts as an oxygen carrier which in turn enhances the oxygen content of your blood and therefore your red blood cells. They contain fibre which helps keep the bowel healthy, an absolute must for a healthy immune system, especially if you're having chemotherapy. Try to eat as much raw veg as possible and don't think this just means eating a normal meal uncooked. There's a whole food movement in raw food preparation these days, it's completely delicious and you would be hard pushed to realise nothing has been cooked.

4. whole fruits and avocados

By this I mean fresh, whole fruits which still contain all the fibre. Try to avoid fruit which has been processed in any way and if you are allowed fruit juice, make sure that you either make your own or buy the best quality fruit juice that you can afford and dilute it with water. Avoid anything labelled 'fruit drink' as this is normally sugar water with a little fruit and fruit flavourings added.

Do check with your nutritionist which fruits are best for you as some are very acidic or very high in sugar, both of which are best to avoid. I tended to stick to fresh pears, pineapples, papaya and the occasional banana. Watermelon was also a welcome addition.

I believe avocado is usually classed as a fruit but whether it's a fruit or a vegetable it is certainly one of the best. It is alkaline, contains many vitamins and minerals and I carry one with me as it's like a complete salad on its own. Not only is it delicious, and nutritious, it can work wonders for your skin.

5. short grain brown rice

This rice is a godsend if you are on a metabolic diet. Although it's a starchy grain, it doesn't release such high amounts of sugar as other grains. It's a great way to bulk up vegetable meals especially when seasoned with a yeast-free stock cube which you can buy in most health food shops these days. Be careful not to keep leftover rice as it can develop microbes that can be harmful, so try to cook it fresh. I find the easiest way to cook it is to use two parts water to one part rice, bring to the boil then reduce heat to a low simmer and cover with a lid. Do not stir it or disturb it but leave until you test a few grains and find them to be tender (about 30 minutes) Blending cooked rice into a soup is also a great thickener and has been a quick option when I've got in from work many times. Instead of grains I use quinoa either as seeds or as flakes and millet flakes. You can also buy millet and quinoa flour, but don't expect them to behave as other flours as they are gluten-free. They are alkaline, low in starch therefore low in sugar and certainly better than nothing. The recipes I've included in this book will give some ideas on how to use these products.

6. nuts and seeds, apricot kernels

Choose fresh, raw nuts. Avoid roasted, salted or any other kind of processed nuts such as dry roasted. Steer clear of peanuts as they can contain microbes which is something to be avoided on a cancer recovery program. Try not to do what I did which was to go mad on eating cashews until I couldn't bear the sight of them for over a year! Make sure that any nuts you eat have no mould even on their shells as this is another form of fungus which you would do well to avoid on this program. They also contain vitamins and minerals such as Zinc (found in Brazil nuts) and Vitamin E (found in walnuts) and, best of all, Vitamin B17 which is most concentrated in apricot kernels. I could write a whole chapter on this alone but, suffice it to say, Vitamin B17 may have the ability to penetrate and destroy some cancer cells and act as a nutrient to healthy cells. Make sure you buy the best quality apricot kernels. I still consume five kernels every day and will always do so. Previously I had bought B17 tablets from the USA but prefer the kernels as they contain other vitamins which enhance absorption.

7. lentils and pulses

Pulses include beans and chickpeas. These are great fillers but check which ones are compatible with your diet. In the meantime you can't really go far wrong using pretty much any beans and lentils. Split peas should be ok, but ordinary garden peas are rather high in sugar. Use dried pulses or cans of organic chickpeas or beans in spring water. If they are in salt water, give them a rinse before using. Some supermarkets do sell canned organic chickpeas and beans.

One of the best products I found was organic chickpea pasta. I virtually lived on this stuff and it still comprises a significant part of my diet. Chickpea pasta behaves pretty much as conventional wheat pasta and you can cook it from frozen. Chickpeas can also be bought as flour, more commonly known as gram flour, which is perfect for onion bhajis.

8. green, white and herbal teas

This is a matter of taste. Again, go for organic whenever possible. As I mentioned before, I'm a big tea drinker and I tend to go for the green and white varieties. I prefer loose teas when I'm at home but have to resort to bags for convenience when I'm on the go. I'm not fond of most herbal teas but having said that I often pick herbs such as sage, thyme, or lavender from my garden in the summer and just dunk them in a cup of hot water. There are a huge amount of health benefits to be had from herbs and I would suggest reading up on this further down the line if you have the inclination. There are also some lovely varieties of tea to choose from in health food shops.

9. onions and garlic herbs and spices

All these are wonderful for providing flavour but they are also packed with powerful antioxidants and vitamins. Garlic contains allicin which is probably one of the best natural cleansers and anti-fungal agents available. Spices such as turmeric are packed with curcumin which is a powerful anti-cancer agent. Checkout the onion bhaji recipe in the recipe section, which uses gram flour, turmeric, salt and onions. Do experiment with herbs and spices to discover flavours which you enjoy.

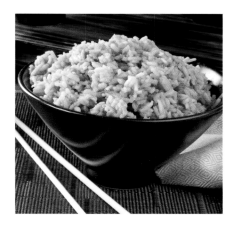

10. fish and meat

Opinions vary on whether we should consume fish and meat when on a cancer recovery programme. Generally speaking, most nutritionists suggest white meat, and deep-sea fish such as cod and haddock, as deep-sea fish is less likely to contain high levels of pollutants than fish from shallower waters or farmed fish. However, some regimes advocate a completely vegan approach which excludes all animal products. Check this out carefully as some cancers can deplete protein which means that protein will be required in the diet. (I got a lot of extra advice about this from Patricia Peat (see the Resources section for her details).

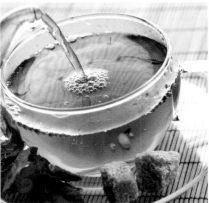

As for me, I'd been a non-meat eater for about thirty five years but I enjoyed any fish except farmed fish as not only has that made me very ill on more than one occasion, it can contain high levels of toxins. I was advised to eat small amounts of wild or organic fish but I reasoned that if I cut back and I recovered, I'd never know if fish was an issue and would always have to be wary of it, so I thought I'd carry on as usual and cut back if things weren't working out. So I carried on with the fresh tuna steaks and after about eighteen months when Dr Andre agreed I could have a few prawns I went out to dinner and had a lobster. Lovely it was too!

I need to stress that you should think about what serves you best in your situation, don't just go about it the way I did.

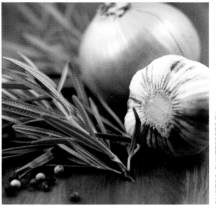

RECIPES

Ten recipes to get you started

I've included recipes for food to take out with you, as you can't always rely on finding something appropriate to eat when you're on the move. I remember going into a theatre with my friend Mitch Murray, a dedicated Foodie, when he commented that he was glad they hadn't searched our bags, as he had a tub of egg mayonnaise and a packet of prosciutto in his. I replied that I was carrying a can of mackerel and an avocado!

Keep all ingredients fresh and organic wherever possible.

It helps to enjoy these recipes for what they are, rather than to see them as a substitute for other dishes. Above all, try to include vegetables wherever possible. If you can't obtain or afford organic, at least make sure your produce is as fresh as possible.

As long as you check that the ingredients you use are admissible for your own programme, feel free to experiment, don't be afraid to play around and you will create some delicious surprises.

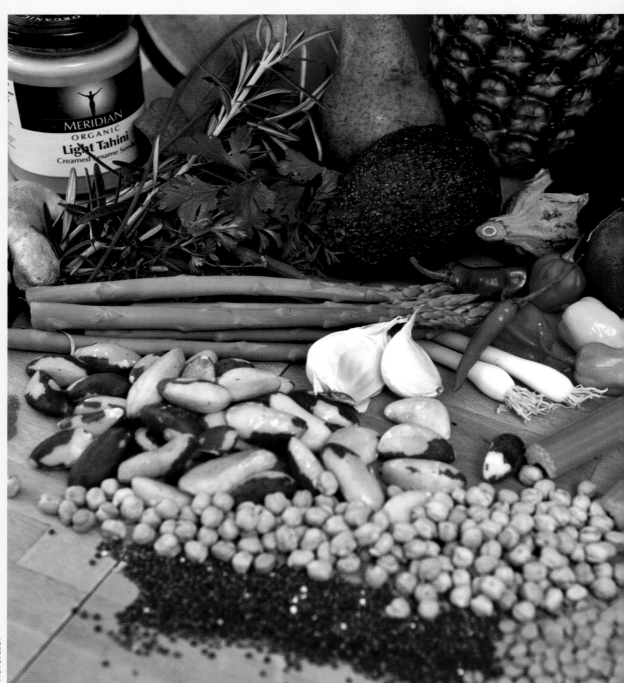

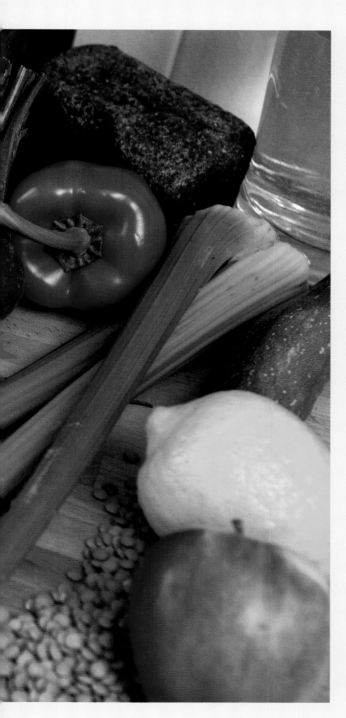

1. onion bhajis

Ingredients
Coconut oil or butter for frying
4 medium onions
3 tbs gram flour
3 teaspoons turmeric
Salt to taste
Lemon and fresh coriander to serve

Method
Place flour, salt and turmeric in a bowl and add chopped or sliced onions, using a little water to bind to a reasonably thick batter, or loose dough.

Heat 1 cm oil in a pan *(Deep frying in olive oil can prove expensive especially as heated oil shouldn't be re-used)* When oil is hot, turn down heat then place separate spoonfuls of onion mixture into the pan and fry until they turn a light brown. Then turn them over and repeat. Place on kitchen paper to blot excess oil. Continue until all the onion batter is used.

Serve immediately garnished with wedges of lemon and coriander.

NB: You can use other vegetables such as broccoli which you may want to blanche first (if you're not used to raw ones) or use lightly cooked vegetables such as spinach or courgettes, instead of onions. An Indian friend of mine said this is the only way she can get her children to eat vegetables.

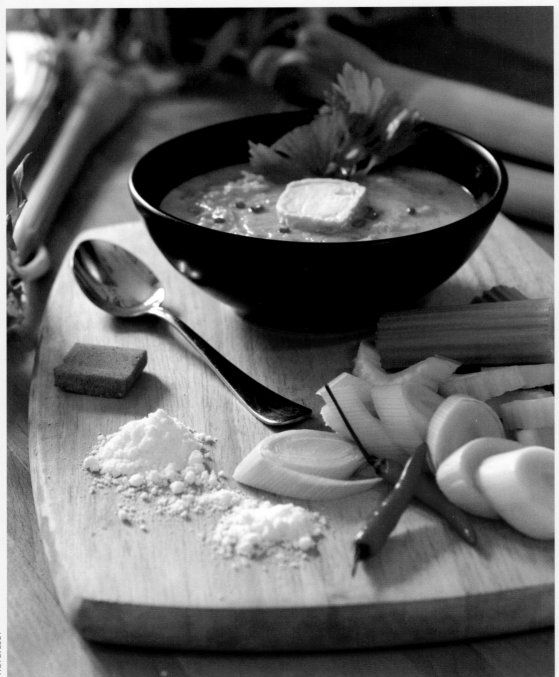

2. celery and coconut soup

makes six generous servings

Ingredients
Knob of butter or coconut oil
1 head of celery
2 leeks or two medium onions
1 fresh red chilli (optional)
½ can of coconut milk (I often buy coconut milk powder, to avoid wasting the other half tin)
1 yeast-free stock cube
Approx 500ml bottled or filtered water

Method
Slice onions or leeks and fry in coconut oil or butter for approximately 2 minutes or until just becoming soft. Cut celery into 1cm slices and finely chop chilli and add to onions or leeks.

Fry for a further two minutes. Pour over the water *(it should sit about an inch lower than the top of the vegetable mixture)* and add one stock cube. Simmer until celery is tender but not overdone *(about five minutes)*. Turn off the heat and place in a blender or use a hand blender and roughly blend leaving some larger pieces. Add coconut milk to taste (usually about half the can). Serve hot.

NB. If you're allowed goats' cheese, a few pieces dropped into each bowl can add another delicious dimension.

3. 'Jessica Sez' pasties

Whilst at Dr Andre's clinic, the other patients were laughing that each time they discussed food it seemed to be preceded with, "Jessica Sez"
The reason I had so much to say about it is because I had been there longer and I'm a natural busybody!

Pastry Ingredients
One part organic coconut oil
Three parts quinoa flour and water to mix

Method
Rub the oil into the flour as with normal pastry until it has a crumbly texture. Gradually add cold water and knead until it forms pastry texture. If you overdo it with the water add more flour (unlike pastries made with ordinary flour this requires a bit more kneading). Let pastry rest at least half an hour before rolling. Then take a small ball of the dough and roll it with the rolling pin *(using quinoa flour to stop it sticking)* to make a circular shape ready for filling. To fill, spoon mixture into centre of circle, dampen edges of circle with water and squeeze together as in a Cornish pasty.

NB: This won't have the stretch of normal pastry, so don't worry if your pasties have got a few cracks or holes, it just adds to their charm!

Suggestions for filling
Practically anything can be used here. One of the best is leftover curry perhaps mixed with some rice. Or make up a mixture of beans, pulses, chickpeas, lentils and vegetables of your choice. Any of these variations work well, especially if you add a yeast-free stock cube to the mixture (if you are allowed it), or some Tamari sauce.

NB: If you're being treated by Dr Andre, watch him if you bring these in because he loves them!

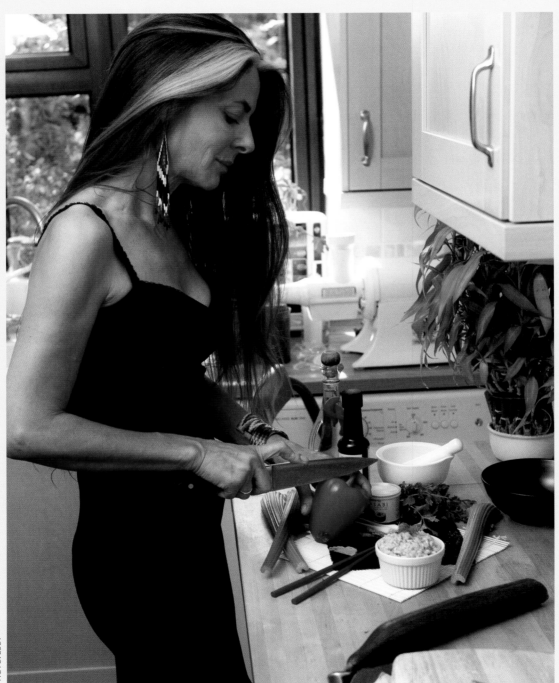

4. chickpea pasta with vegetables

Serves 2 – 4 depending on portion size

Ingredients

1 large onion
1 courgette
1 small head of broccoli
1 medium bunch of fresh spinach or two portions of frozen
½ cup of fresh or frozen peas
1 can of organic plum tomatoes
Dried or fresh basil and / or thyme to taste
1 large squeeze of organic tomato puree
Few sprigs of fresh parsley for serving

(You can vary vegetables according to preference or availability)

Method

Fry onions in coconut oil or butter until soft. Cut broccoli and courgettes into approx. 2 cm pieces. Add courgettes and broccoli to onion mixture and cook until almost soft enough, adding a little water if necessary.

Add peas and tear up spinach if fresh or add frozen portions. Add rock salt or pink Himalayan salt to taste, with the can of organic, plum tomatoes. Then cook the chickpea pasta as directed on the packet. Add herbs to the vegetable mix, taste, and simmer for a few minutes while adding the tomato puree. Pour the sauce over the pasta, or mix in and serve immediately sprinkled with a little fresh parsley.

5. polenta with sun dried tomatoes, shitake mushrooms and fresh herbs

Serves 2 – 3

Ingredients

1 pack of prepared polenta
(available from supermarkets) You can make it from scratch, I buy dried organic polenta from my health food shop as it's easy to make and at least I know it's not made from genetically modified maize.
1 punnet of shitake mushrooms
(available from most supermarkets)
About 3 sun-dried tomatoes
Handful of mixed fresh herbs such as sage, coriander, or thyme
Garlic if desired
Knob of butter or permitted fat or oil for frying

Method

Heat butter or oil in shallow frying pan. Slice mushrooms *(and garlic if used)* and fry in the butter or oil for 1 minute. Cut the polenta into 1cm thick slices and add to the mushrooms. Immediately cut up tomatoes and add to polenta and mushrooms. Cook on low heat until polenta is hot through, turning once. Finally, tear up the herbs and add to the rest. Serve hot.

NB: This can be a great breakfast dish served with a couple of poached eggs.

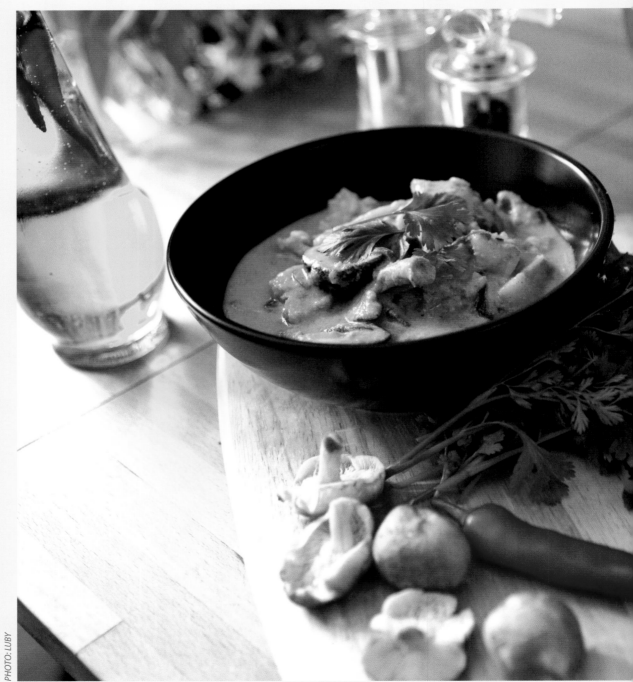

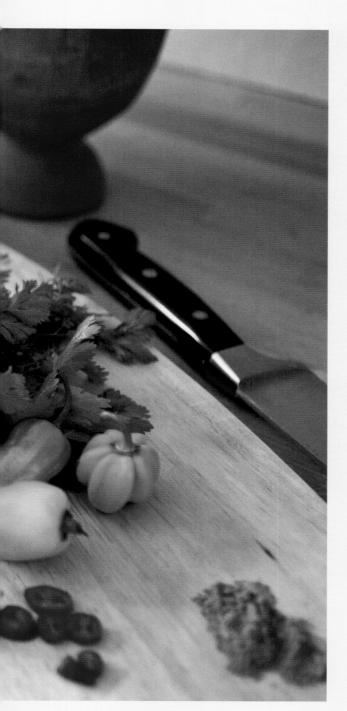

6. Wendy's curry

A version of this curry was made by my sister Wendy when our mother was ill and was our mother's favourite dish.

Ingredients
1 chilli
Clove garlic
2cms piece of root ginger
2 tsp turmeric
2 organic chicken breasts, cubed
1 pack shitake mushrooms
Half cup of organic rice flour
½ can organic coconut milk
1 organic, yeast-free stock cube
Bunch fresh coriander
Butter or coconut oil for frying

Method
Fry ginger, garlic and chilies in the coconut oil or organic salted butter. *(Take care not to breathe in fumes when you add the chilli as it can sting your nose and throat)*. Add the chicken pieces coated in organic rice flour until brown and sealed. Add coconut milk, turmeric and stock cube with a little water and bring to the boil. Add mushrooms *(sliced)* and simmer until chicken is cooked. *(About six minutes)*. When cooked, garnish with the chopped fresh coriander *(optional)*. Serve with boiled short grain brown rice *(one part rice to two parts water, bring to boil then turn to very low heat until tender)*

OR : alternatively serve with your own choice of fresh, steamed organic vegetables, or substitute fish for the chicken.

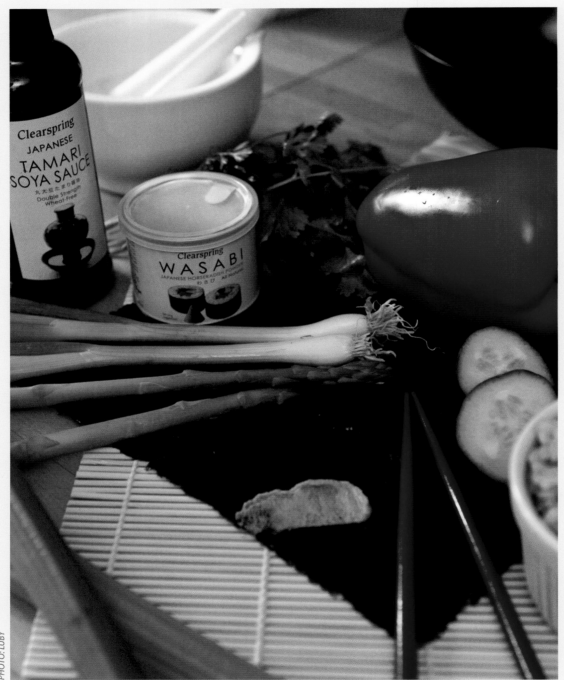

PHOTO: LUBY

7. vegetarian sushi

This was a favourite of Dr Lynette Yong, and many times we'd nearly blow our heads off with the wasabi sauce.

Ingredients

1 Packet of Nori seaweed sheets
(available from healthfood shops and most supermarkets)
1 cup short grain brown rice
½ cucumber
½ each of red, green and yellow pepper
2 spring onions
These are suggestions, you can use any vegetables of your choice

Tamari soy sauce and Wasabi paste to serve

Method

Put cup of rice in saucepan with two cups of cold bottled or filtered water and bring to the boil. Turn down the heat and simmer with the lid on for around 20 minutes or until rice is tender (You can add a yeast-free stock cube but it's fine without). While the rice is cooking, thinly slice the vegetables. Allow the cooked rice to cool down. Lay out one sheet of Nori seaweed and place some rice around 2cms from the near edge. Place a small bunch of the sliced vegetables on top of the rice and roll the seaweed around it as if rolling a cigarette. Seal the edge with a little water to keep it closed. Continue until you have enough, then take a sharp knife and cut into 2 – 3cm lengths. Serve with the Tamari and Wasabi. Keep in a sealed container in the fridge and eat within 24hrs.

8. thick vegetable soup

6+ servings

This is a great standby, or is perfect if you have friends round for a casual gathering such as a bonfire or firework party.

Ingredients

1 large onion
1 large floret of broccoli
1 red pepper
2 courgettes
1 large handful of spinach
1 chilli *(optional)*
1 tablespoon of short grain rice
up to 2 yeast-free stock cubes
1 teaspoon turmeric
Any allowed or preferred vegetables may be used

Method

Heat some permitted oil or butter in a large saucepan. Slice the onions and fry for a couple of minutes until a little soft then reduce heat. Add turmeric. Break up broccoli florets and add to onions. Boil 1 litre of bottled or filtered water and pour over onions. Add rice and 1 stock cube and leave to cook on a medium heat in the covered pan until tender *(about 30 minutes)*. Slice and add the courgettes and peppers or vegetables of choice. When the vegetables are tender, taste and add more stock cube if desired. Roughly blend with a hand blender.

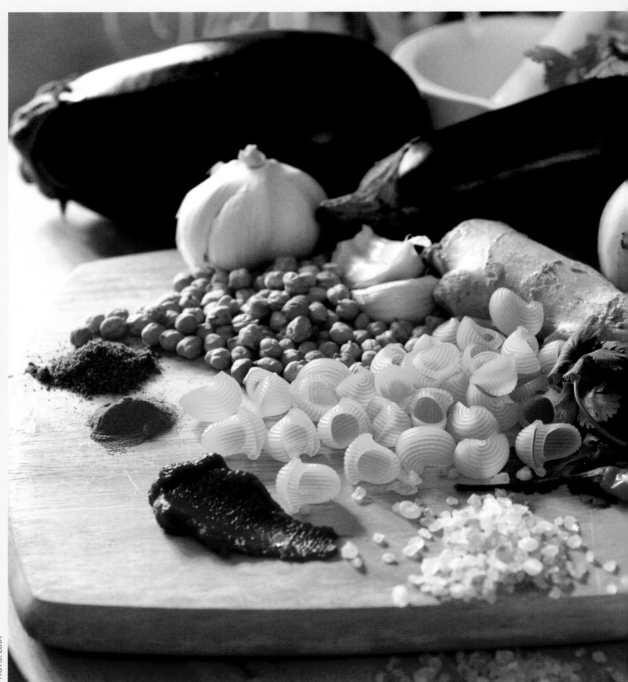

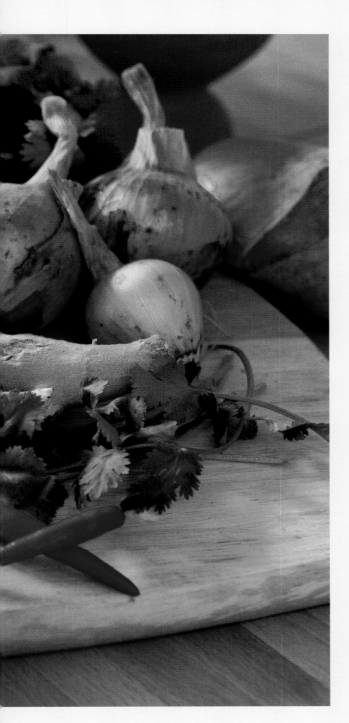

9. *chickpea curry*

This recipe is adapted from Healing Curries by Monisha Bharadwaj. I made it for my friend Tracey when she had the flu and she said she could actually feel its warmth and healing as she ate it.

Ingredients

2 tablespoons of coconut oil
2 medium onions finely sliced
1 clove of garlic crushed
2 cms fresh root ginger finely chopped
1 teaspoon turmeric powder
1 teaspoon ground coriander
1 red chilli finely chopped
Pink Himalayan salt to taste
1 medium aubergine cut into 2.5cms (1") pieces, or small head of broccoli
200g tinned organic chickpeas, drained
2 tablespoons fresh coriander leaves finely chopped
2 tablespoons tomato puree
Around 1 handful of corn pasta or polenta

Method

Heat one tablespoon of oil in a heavy-based saucepan and fry the onions over a high heat until soft *(about five minutes)*. Add the ginger, garlic and tomato puree and fry until mushy. Add the chilli. Cool slightly and then transfer the ingredients to a blender or use a hand blender and blitz to a smooth puree adding a little water if necessary. Put to one side and use the pan to heat the remaining oil. Add the aubergine and powdered spices and stir-fry for about 1 minute to coat the aubergine in the oil and spices. Add the mixture from the blender and season with salt. Pour in 100ml of water and bring to the boil stirring all the time. Add the pasta or polenta and the chickpeas.

Reduce the heat and cover with a lid and cook for 8 minutes or until pasta is cooked and aubergine is tender. Garnish with the fresh coriander.

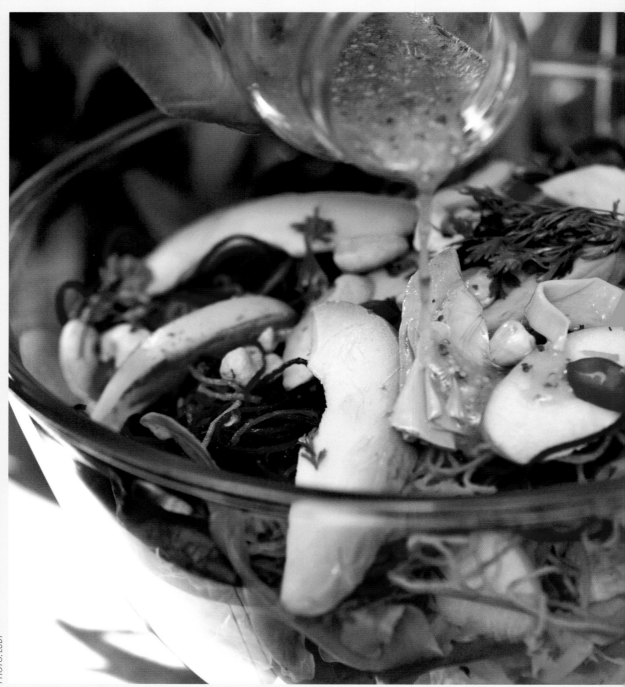

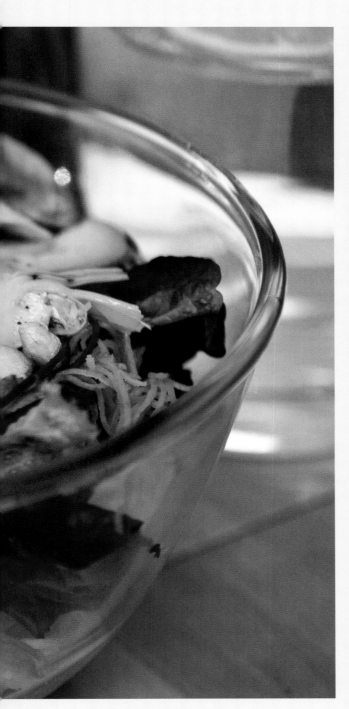

10. Jessica's favourite salad

I like to eat a huge salad every day. If I don't, I actually begin to get cravings. This one has a lot of variety and is very filling.

Ingredients
Salad leaves
Shredded or grated raw carrot and beetroot
Sprouting seeds
½ apple
Small chilli *(optional)*
½ avocado
Handful of raw cashews
Whole sun dried tomato
Artichoke hearts

Dressing
I make dressing in a screw top jar and keep it in the fridge. You will need to experiment with proportions to make it to your own taste.

Olive oil
Cider vinegar or lemon juice
Grain mustard
Fresh herbs of choice

Method
Place leaves in a bowl or on a pasta plate. Pile on the carrot and beetroot. Add the remaining ingredients and pour over the dressing

quinoa chapatis

Ingredients
6 tablespoons of quinoa flour
Cold water to bind

Method
Place the flour in a bowl. Gradually add the water as you start kneading. Continue until you make a stiff dough. (If you add too much water, simply add more flour or vice versa. Remember that gluten free flour is less stretchy and requires more kneading). Make a nice round ball and leave to rest for at least 30 minutes. Then flour a surface with quinoa flour. Break off a small piece of dough about the size of a small egg, and knead it in the palm of your hand with a bit more flour. Roll it into a ball then, using a rolling pin, roll into a circle around 2mm thick. Keep going until you've used up the dough or made the desired amount.

To cook, heat a dry frying pan on a high heat. When hot, place chapatti in for 30 seconds then turn over and cook the other side in the same way. Serve hot with soups and curries, or cold as wraps for salad or any filling of your choice. If using cold, try to make the wraps just prior to eating as they can go soft and break up over time.

I found it very useful to keep a supply of these in the fridge. To do this, flour a plate and place a layer of flour between each uncooked chapatti, cover and keep in fridge and use as required. Eat within three days. Alternatively, if you cook them first, they'll keep in an airtight container for up to five days.

chickpea mash

Ingredients
Can of organic chickpeas
Two table spoons of olive oil
Clove of garlic
Half a yeast free stock cube
Mixed herbs of choice

Method
Blend all the ingredients together until they are a smooth mash. Fry with a little coconut oil in a hot pan until brown on both sides (five -six minutes) and serve hot in place of potatoes. Instead of herbs, you can use a teaspoon of curry powder and fresh chopped chilli to taste, or a pinch of chilli powder.

hummus

You can use this on crackers or biscuits, and I've often used it to dress salad. Although it's thick, it gives the salad some 'body'. It's also good used as a spread instead of butter.

Ingredients
1 can of organic chickpeas (You may want to get into the finer points of using dried and soaking and sprouting before use but for now, here's the quick version)
2 tablespoons of tahini
Juice of 1 – 1 ½ lemons
Approx 3 tablespoons of extra virgin olive oil
3 cloves of garlic
Freshly ground black pepper to taste

Method
Blend all ingredients together adding oil until preferred consistency. Keep refrigerated in an airtight container and use within a few days.

broad bean summer pate

This is quick and easy to make and will keep in the fridge for a few days. It's ideal for snacks and also makes a wonderful accompaniment to fish or chicken and vegetable dishes.

Ingredients

500gms fresh broad beans, or canned if fresh aren't available. I try to avoid canned or preserved if possible by using seasonal ingredients. Hence, I tend to make this with fresh beans in the summer months when they are freely available
1 tablespoon olive oil
Juice of ½ lemon *(or lime if permitted)*
1 clove garlic
1 red chilli *(to taste)*
Ground black pepper to taste
Himalayan pink salt to taste
Pinch of smoked paprika for garnish

Method

Lightly steam beans *(about three minutes)* Remove from heat and place in bowl. Add all of the oil then the remainder of ingredients in increments whilst beans are still hot and blend with a hand blender. Keep adding remaining ingredients until desired taste and consistency. Turn into serving bowl garnished with the smoked paprika. Serve warm or cold with crackers, rice cakes, sprouted hemp bread etc. with extra lemon to squeeze if desired.

avocado and lemon salad dressing

Blend an avocado with a clove of garlic, juice of a lemon and about two teaspoons of olive oil, and toss with salad.

pineapple and herb salad dressing

Juice fresh organic pineapple *(if you are allowed it)*, mix with a small clove of crushed garlic and fresh herbs such as parsley, thyme or mint, and toss with salad.

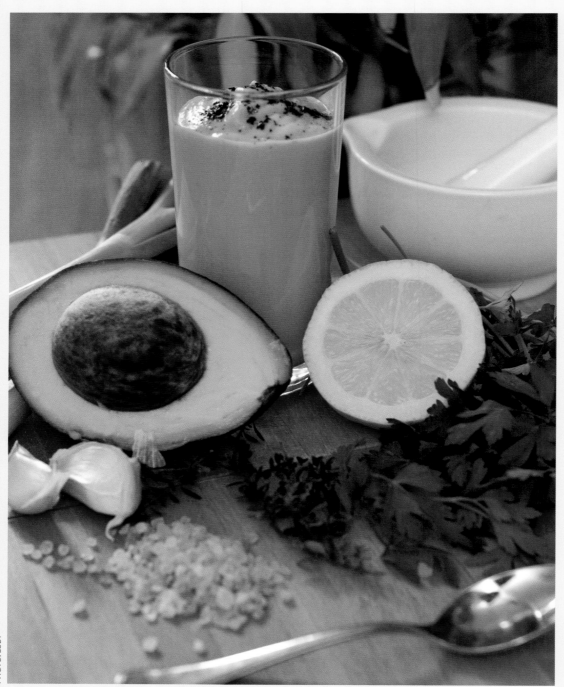

avocado smoothie

This is very useful and can be used as a savoury cold soup. These are basic ingredients but do experiment, not only for your own taste but to support your own recovery program as there are some ingredients which can be very helpful if you are undergoing radiotherapy or chemotherapy.

Ingredients
1 ripe avocado
Lemon juice to blend
1 spring onion
Small clove of garlic
Sprig of parsley and/or fresh thyme.
Pinch of Himalayan pink salt
1 tablespoon of linseed oil

Method
Place all the ingredients in blender and blend until smooth. Otherwise use a hand blender.
(You can also add things like chlorella tablets or spirulina if these are a part of your programme.)

spiced spinach or greens

Adapted from Premila Lal's Indian Cooking for Pleasure

This is a great way to serve greens and makes a change from just steaming.

Ingredients
2 large onions
½' fresh ginger root
2 cloves garlic
2 tomatoes
2lb spinach or other greens
Coconut oil or butter for frying.
2 cloves
1 cardamom seed
1 teaspoon chilli powder (Optional)
1 teaspoon garam masala
Himalayan pink salt to taste

Method
Finely cut onions into rings and finely chop or mince ginger. Wash the spinach and cook in pan until tender without adding any water. *(If using greens, slice and lightly steam)* Drain and puree *(I use a hand blender for this)*. Heat a little oil and fry the onions, ginger and garlic for two minutes. Add cloves and cardamom and fry for another minute. Put in the tomatoes and fry for a further three minutes. Then add chilli powder *(if using)* and garam masala. Simmer until liquid has evaporated *(around ten minutes)*. Stir in the puree and season with salt. Serve hot with fish, boiled eggs, chicken etc.

my 'nearest you can get to dessert'

If you're sticking to this diet, you're probably gagging for a dessert by now so this should help.

Toast two slices of organic sprouted hemp or rye bread, or wrap them in foil and warm in the oven. Warm some tahini by standing the jar in a bowl of hot water, pour over the bread and on top of that, drizzle a little bit of agave syrup (if allowed it) to taste. It tastes great with syrup but pretty good without. Try adding a few slices of banana or pears depending on your particular diet.

baked pears with cinnamon

The clue here is in the title. Most diets will include hard, UK fruit such as pears and apples as they're lower in sugar.

Ingredients
1-2 under ripe pears per person
Sprinkling of cinnamon
Agave syrup if allowed

Method
Peel the pears, cut into quarters or halves and remove the cores. Place in a shallow dish. Drizzle over a little syrup if using. Sprinkle liberally with ground cinnamon. Place in a pre-heated oven at 180°, until pears are tender, turning them once. Serve hot, warm or cold as preferred.

My basic ingredient checklist

This is a good list to get you started. All ingredients are available in good health food shops and some supermarkets.

Quinoa grains, flour and flakes*
Millet flour and flakes *
Gram flour *#
Coconut milk. *#
Canned or dried organic lentils *#
Canned or dried organic chickpeas *#
Short grain brown rice. *
Yeast-free stock cubes. *
Stevia and / or agave syrup *
Sprouted hemp / rye bread *
Olive oil #
Flax oil. *#
Rice milk *#
Nut milk *#
Oat milk *#
Coconut oil (food quality) *#
Nuts (except peanuts) *#
Seeds. *#
Organic tomato puree and canned tomatoes #
Herbs and spices *#
Tamari soy sauce *#
Wasabi paste *#
Tahini *#
Pink Himalayan salt. *
Polenta *#

Fresh produce
Garlic
Onions
Chillies
Greens and salad
Cucumbers (for salads and juicing)
Lemons
Wheatgrass tray
Organic chickpea pasta *#
1 large box of determination and imagination!
(You already have that)

My basic equipment checklist:

juicer

There are many available, so don't waste time getting too involved with this, it can be time consuming and expensive. Just buy a simple one and get using it! You can look into the more specialised versions when you have experience and more time.

blender

The same is true. You can get very involved in the various aspects of blending and blenders can get very expensive, but initially, just get a simple blender and use it. I actually manage with just a hand blender. (Non-specialised blenders and juicers are available in many retail outlets)

One woman called me because she'd been diagnosed with breast cancer and was eager to put into practice the diet and nutrition aspect of her treatment plan. I was dismayed to receive a second call from her, over two weeks later, to be told that she still hadn't even begun as she was deliberating, amongst other things over which juicer to get. I told her in no uncertain terms that she wasn't buying a new dress or a new car and should not waste any more time! She got the point. Denial can be a funny thing.

available in health food shops
 # available in supermarkets

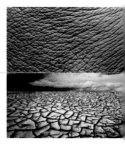

CHAPTER 5

I don't feel very positive, does that mean I won't make it?

Ten ways to change your mind: How to develop the mental discipline to help you recover.

It's not what life presents to us that defines who we are but who we choose to be in relationship to it.

No. If you don't feel very positive, it doesn't mean you'll die. Nobody feels very positive when they've just been diagnosed with cancer. What follows, will show you how you can change that state of mind.

Recently there was a TV series presented by a scientist who investigated various types of treatments, medications, vitamins and so on. Several times during the series many things were written off as merely having a placebo effect, with the inference that a placebo was worthless. Hello? Wasn't there an elephant in the room here? Some great, big, obvious truth that wasn't being acknowledged? Surely a placebo effect, being the power of the mind to bring about a result promised by a drug, treatment or vitamin was worthy of more investigation than being written off in favour of concentrating on the pills, potions or lotions. Babies and bath water come to mind!

It has been my experience that, as far as recovery is concerned, mental discipline is top of the list followed by diet and nutrition, and then treatment. Whatever alternative treatment one looks at, (and many medical practitioners will agree with this) these are the three elements which appear in all cases. Mental discipline is far more important than simply 'positive thinking' or 'belief'. It is a definite decision to recover, followed by behaviour which demonstrates that decision. *This is vitally important. Make your decision, then commit to it and act out that commitment in your behaviour.*

Most people avail themselves of conventional or alternative treatment based purely on belief, going ahead without question in the belief that they will be cured. Lots of positive people who believe in what they're doing still don't make it, but don't be concerned. This chapter will enable you to develop the mental discipline that can enhance your recovery and enable you to make sound decisions based on relevant information and clear thinking. This is where my many years of training and practice in hypnotherapy and self-development really came into play. Some people may have a more positive attitude than others but let me assure you that mental discipline can be developed so don't be concerned if you think you just weren't made that way.

Here's how I did it. It's not easy but it is simple. You will need to concentrate and force yourself to keep your mind in the present and not allow it to wander off into the realm of nightmares. I remember reading somewhere that yes, I could die from cancer but I have no intention of dying every day worrying about it!

Much of modern medical practice is based on the 'belief' that the mind and the body are separate entities. Just because it is a belief doesn't make it the truth.

Ten ways to change your mind and develop the mental discipline to recover.

1.   Accept the situation and make a decision.

First, accept the situation. I mean the *facts* of the situation, not hearsay or imagination. Then make a definite decision to stay alive, followed by an informed plan. I know that armed response officers in the police force, the military and other emergency workers when facing a life threatening situation are trained, to decide to stay alive, and to tell themselves or the person they are helping that they will live. This has been proved to increase survival rates in such situations dramatically. Really commit to your decision to stay alive. It should feel like a decision and not just a hope or wish. Even if it starts out as a hope or wish, keep acting as though it is a decision and it will soon feel like one.

2.   Accept the facts, don't get involved in the story.

Accept the facts fully but don't get involved in the story. Make sure you deal with the facts as they apply to you. For instance, if the fact is that the cancer you're dealing with has a 70% fatality rate don't take this personally and translate it as, you have a 70% chance of dying. Not so. Although the figures show that 70% of people may die

from that cancer, a) you may be one of the 30% who has a 100% chance of recovery, and b) you may have a different mindset and different treatment from other people in the study. Remember, as I wrote in Chapter One, some medical data seems to be based on very little input.

We seem to have a situation where some people will die no matter what treatment is given and others recover despite seemingly bleak odds against them. I couldn't take the results of the kind of data I was offered as scientific fact, because so many other aspects such as mental attitude, social and financial circumstances (we know that generally speaking, the poor die younger than the rich!) spiritual beliefs, dietary habits and so on, are not taken into account. Bear this in mind when reviewing the facts of your own situation.

The facts in my case were: I had a breast tumour of approximately 3.5cms. It was not known whether it was in my lymph and without knowing any more than this at the time, there was no way of having any idea what my chances of survival were. I had no clear idea as to how I got cancer. These were the facts at the time. The story, on the other hand was ' I've got cancer!' I might die, how painful will it be? I live a long way from my family, shall I have my funeral near them or where I live? What will happen to Alan? What about the cats? What if I have chemotherapy, I'll look like Ghandi! I could still be bald when I die. If I don't die, my hair will grow back white and if I grow it as long as it is, I'll have to invest in a black pointed hat! I can't let my parents see me go through the suffering of that treatment. Shall I stay away and not tell them? Will that be worse for them? If I lose my hair everyone will know I've got cancer, I'm not young enough to pass it off as a fashion statement!'

And the worst of it all for me was, "I'll have to hand my life over to the system." The thought of that alone was enough to make my hair fall out! (It did occur to me that I'd always wanted to have enough money to last me the rest of my life and I thought, what a bummer that it could come true, not because I'd become rich but because I could be running out of life! Talk about be careful what you wish for!)

So you see, the story can go on forever and is not a good place to be. I forced myself to focus only on the facts and deal with them. At least this way I had some power. I listed the facts and dealt with them one at a time, always keeping my mind focussed in the present. Literally *act* with Presence of Mind. I chose to have a lymph node biopsy first, in order to find out if it had spread to the lymph as, until I knew this, it wasn't possible to make any other decisions, apart from deciding to tell others only on a need to know basis.

3.   Choose your team.

It doesn't have to be a large team (although it may expand over time). It can be made up of just one or two people. Quality is the important thing so be discerning and make sure that, above all, the people you choose support you fully in the treatment you choose. Even if you haven't decided on a treatment yet, it's essential that you pick people who will support you personally no matter what. If you choose alternative treatment, don't be disappointed or upset if your team doesn't include your family. It's not always possible for those who love you to support you in something they don't believe in, especially as their opinions are likely to be based on fear rather than information. Most people believe that if you follow the 'normal' route, at least it will soon all be over and done with. Few people who've been through it will agree with that!

Here's how my team evolved:

Firstly, I had my partner Alan, the first to be told and who supported me unconditionally. He was also a voice of calm and reason whenever I was shouting the odds about something or other. Then I told my friend and neighbour Astrid, who kept my other neighbours informed. Her positive and cheerful attitude and commitment to learning what she could about my diet enabled me to join in with the usual social functions with our other friends and neighbours. (Astrid and I also went out dancing together regularly!)

My GP was a key member of my team. He listened patiently to my rantings and wrote many letters of referral to the specialists I wanted to see, whilst at the same time, pleading with me not to leave things too long before I did something physically.

I told my friend Marisa, who took me into her home to take care of me before the lymph node surgery and was by my side for many of my other appointments as well. She was a mine of information and was a great help with various research. Then came Phillip Day who was not only available for me to talk to several times a week and on whose research and experience I based much of my treatment plan, but he also gave me the contact details of doctors who could help me. From these, I chose Dr Andre Young Snell, to take care of all of my alternative treatments.

Next came my father 'Chuck', who never doubted my ability to make the right decisions and never questioned the choices I made. I was never in any doubt of his love and respect for me.

Then Mr Kissin, to oversee all medical aspects of my treatments (blood tests, scans and so on).

My friend Dr Lynette Yong professionally liaised with Dr Andre to develop my hormonal treatment plan as well as supporting me with her friendship, and my friend Brenda Golding supported me spiritually as well as with her excellent therapies of polarity healing and reflexology.

Then I talked to Alan's mother Sheila who took me into her home whilst I was being treated at Dr Andre's clinic and helped me develop recipes using the ingredients from Dr Andre's anti-cancer diet plan. Sheila was born in an era when everyone was taught basic cooking skills so she was more easily able to adapt recipes to the allowable ingredients.

So you see, each person became involved in their own capacity and contributed what they were best qualified to give. When you have cancer everyone wants to help and they can help, it's just a matter of finding how they can be of most help to you.

Your team may consist of just one or two people, or it may evolve as mine did, to include many more. I know that if you take a conventional route you will have access to a consultant, radiologist and a cancer nurse, so it's worth making use of them in their own capacity. There are also charities such as Macmillan and Marie Curie, who have many systems of support on offer.

4.   Surround yourself with positive people.

Surround yourself, and interact with positive people wherever possible. If you find there is anyone in your life who is pessimistic or has a negative attitude or who simply can't help recounting all the cancer stories they know, ditch them! I know this sounds a bit harsh but you are in a life and death situation and you can't afford to indulge these types. You may also wish to factor in the temperament of your consultant here. I'm sure that in the not-too-distant future patients and consultants' personalities, values and attitudes will be taken into account when allocating patients to a consultant.

If you can't avoid such people because you have to live or work with them, make sure that you have an antidote, someone you can call or have a cup of tea with. I was most grateful to have Dr Andre and the other patient of his who had been through the same treatment. I was actually relieved when she told me that she also went through bad days during her recovery. I was also glad to be able to speak with Phillip Day for a top up on the facts.

5.   Remain present.

Keeping yourself focussed in the present also means paying close attention to everything else that's going on around you. Really pay attention to day-to-day events and conversations. Look at the sky, enjoy your children, literally smell the roses. Just pay attention to where you are right now.

I remember right at the beginning, I met a friend, Julia, for lunch. We had a long conversation and she reminded me about staying present and being grateful for each moment. It was just what I needed to hear at the time, as everything was looming so bleak and frightening. In fact I'd just had a meeting with a business colleague who was already planning who I should hand my business clients on to! On my way back to the Angel tube station, I came across a young man, who I think was selling something. I was concentrating on remaining completely present and in that moment. As I approached he smiled broadly, and opened his arms. I walked into them and we just laughed and hugged. He wished me well and I went into the station, grateful that I'd been present enough not to miss that moment. I don't know what was going through his mind and nor do I care, it was just a spontaneous thing that happened in the moment. I can't guarantee that sort of thing will happen to you but you'll never know if you don't pay attention will you?

You need to concentrate. Force yourself to keep your mind on the situation in hand, don't allow it to wander off into the realm of nightmares. If you worry about the whole thing, it can be overwhelming, I compared dealing with cancer to eating an elephant, it can seem a bit daunting if you look at the whole thing, so just deal with it one bite at a time.

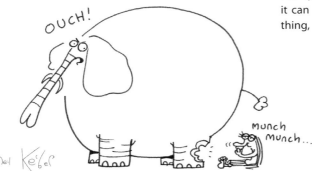

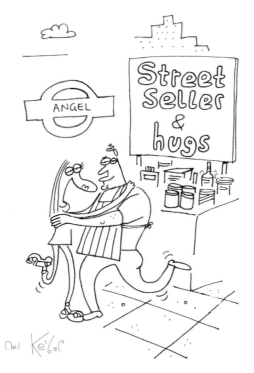

6.   Focus on recovery not survival.

To me, the feel of these two words is very different. 'Survivor' smacks of 'victim' someone who made it by the skin of her teeth. As far as I'm concerned, whether I lived or died, I was in no way a victim, nor would I allow myself to feel like one.

On the other hand, compare that to the word 'Recovery'. How much more powerful it feels. Don't worry if you can't believe that about yourself yet, just act as you would if you were recovering and the feeling will follow. This is the general rule when developing mental discipline. Don't wait to *feel* in a certain way before you begin *acting* in a certain way, decide on the desired outcome and begin to act it immediately, indefatigably, and relentlessly while remaining present. You will then begin to experience the enthusiasm which is the driver, the life force. Words are very powerful things. Choose yours carefully, and this includes the words you think!

7.   Two types of denial – know the difference.

It's common to believe that being in denial is a bad thing but this may not be the case:

Type A - Here, a person will deny, even to himself or herself, the situation they are facing. I've seen people in advanced stages of cancer still insisting that it's simply a 'healing crisis', and that it's normal when using some alternative treatments, as things will get worse before they get better. I've also seen this same situation where someone is trying to convince him or herself that although the cancer drugs they were taking have disabled them, it was worth it because it at least meant they wouldn't get cancer again. Both types get worse and worse rather than accepting that what they've chosen isn't working, and re-evaluating their treatment plan.

Type B - The other version of denial is when someone fully realises and accepts their situation, and then refuses to allow it to interfere with their life. This fits in with my own attitude. I told more than one consultant that I was not interested in survival, I was interested in living but I wasn't prepared to go to endless lengths to hang on to life at any price. Especially when I was told that I couldn't afford to cut corners, and that chemotherapy, surgery, radiotherapy and so on were the only way through.

I believe the difference between these two types of denial is acceptance. To me, that means accepting the situation, deciding to live, then moving on. Not, accepting the situation then giving up.

8.   What you resist persists and what you face disappears.

This is related to acceptance. Ever been in a situation where you've been told not to laugh and suddenly you feel a compulsion to do it, even though you don't know what you're laughing at? Well, that's an example of 'what you resist, persists'.

I remember a situation years ago, when I was about 20 years old. I was working as a pattern cutter and designer at a leather couturier which also did a brisk trade in kinky outfits. One of these outfits was a fitted leather hood and, not having experience in making patterns for such things, the lady who ran the workroom said I should come in when the client was being fitted to show me how the pattern should work, to get the right proportions and fit. In order to hide his identity, the client would already be wearing the hood. Just before we went in she turned to me and said, "Whatever happens don't laugh." The thought hadn't crossed my mind until that point but I knew I had to make sure I stood behind him facing her. She went through agonies looking at my crumpled face whilst having to keep a straight face herself. She knew as well as I did that it would've been fine if she hadn't said that to me just before we went in!

I applied this principle to cancer, and instead of trying to deny it or to avoid thinking about it I focussed on it calmly, but deliberately. There is something special about focusing your attention onto something.

I remember when I was 12 years old, I'd burned my right thumb and the pain would only abate if I held it in a cup of water. When I went to bed that evening, I tried lying on my front with my thumb in the cup of water, which I'd placed on a chair next to my bed. It was impossible to sleep like this and I started to think about why my thumb should still be so painful when it was no longer being burned. I took it out of the water and concentrated on the pain. I focussed my attention on it telling it to do its worst. At first the pain became extremely intense but after a short while, it reduced to one point which felt like a bee sting and then, before I knew it, the point just spiralled off the tip of my thumb which became completely comfortable, as if it had never been burned in the first place.

I used a similar process when concentrating on the tumour. My attitude became calm but intense with the thought, "Kill me or Bog off!"

9. Decide who you are.

We may not be able to predict or choose everything that happens to us, but we can consciously choose who we are in relation to any given situation. When we are clear about who we are, making decisions, even life and death decisions, becomes simple.

During the process of considering various treatments, especially conventional treatments with their potentially serious side effects, I really had to be sure of who I was in order to make decisions. For instance, I choose to be a very physical person. I find great joy in experiencing life through a very fit and healthy body. I like to run and I like to dance and spend a lot of my time doing both. For me there is nothing quite like the feeling of being able to run for a train, across platforms and up and down stairs without becoming breathless. Or to jive dance for hours and hardly break a sweat. I like to live most areas of my life at high speed. I also choose to take full responsibility for my own circumstances and take an active interest in all that is going on around me (I can be a bit 'in your face' if the truth be known, a Pollyanna on speed) When considering Tamoxifen for example, where there was a high probability that I would develop osteoporosis as well as some other rather unpleasant side effects, I had to weigh this up with who I am. Could 'Pollyanna on speed' live with osteoporosis? No thanks. That's a price I was not prepared to pay on the off-chance it might improve my chances of survival from a conventional point of view.

The main question is: Who am I, in relation to being diagnosed with cancer? Am I someone who will allow it to intimidate me and will I just allow myself to be processed without question? Or am I someone who will keep possession of myself, make thorough investigations and work through it in a practical way? I chose to be the latter. Success for me is not being alive, but living or dying on my own terms.

Don't allow yourself to be reduced to a mere cancer patient. Do not allow that to become your identity. This is a really important point. There are so many people being diagnosed with cancer (currently one in three and rising) and in breast cancer alone, there are over 40,000 new cases in the UK, and every year the system has to be built up to meet increasing volume. It is very easy therefore to become one of the statistics and no longer an individual. You may notice the references to 'cancer patients' in the press (well, how else can they refer to us?) But it's imperative that you don't start thinking of yourself as only that. You are an individual human being who has developed a disease, of which there are many types.

The fact is that no two cancers are the same. Even cancers of the same type such as breast or prostate or bowel cancer still vary from person to person, so it's important to remember yourself as an individual and if you wish to be treated like one then you must individuate yourself. By this I mean that *you* should decide who's the best consultant for you, or the best cancer nurse or the best alternative clinic and *you* must investigate whether the treatment on offer is right for you at the time.

I remember another person describing how her consultant told her the team would discuss her case and decide the best course of treatment for her. Then they would discuss this with her at the next appointment. My friend said she felt kind of 'special' that these experts would be conferring to decide a personal plan for her treatment. Their decision was duly discussed on her next hospital visit and she left with a handful of leaflets describing her programme. She braced herself, and began to read through it and realised it was pre-printed and what's more, it was word-for-word what the consultant had just told her! She wondered how she could've been so naive to think that she was special and would be treated as an individual!

This can happen in alternative as well as conventional treatment situations. It's all too easy to get lost in the cancer scenario but you must remember who you are and not allow yourself to be labelled and 'processed' accordingly. That way you can remain in control and keep everything in perspective. You will also be able to be more discerning when choosing your course of treatment and avoid going along with the herd. There's nothing wrong with going along with the herd of course, as long as you've investigated it thoroughly and decided it's the right way for you.

Remember, health professionals are there to take care of your health. Without your input, they have no choice but to make decisions for you.

10. Trust your own intuition.

Remember that you have within you a supreme intelligence that knows what to do and how to do it. It keeps your heart beating and your lungs breathing. If you've ever cut yourself, this part of your mind heals it perfectly, creating all the new cells without any assistance from your conscious mind. There is not one single cell in your body created by drugs. So it stands to reason that we already possess the means to heal ourselves.

I was first aware of my own intuition when my first consultant discussed chemotherapy with me. The very core of my body began to tremble, far beyond the initial fear I was consciously aware of feeling. On my second meeting with him the feeling was even more pronounced and I felt it quite separate from my thoughts about it. I recognised that my own body was in revulsion. It was as sure as it is when you think of eating or drinking something which has previously made you ill, it's a definite physical reaction only much stronger.

Another thing I've done for many years is keep a dream diary. In it, I record dreams and over the years I've written certain questions in my diary and have received the answer via a dream. This is just another way to access your own intuition. Over time I've learned to tell the difference between nonsense dreams, which are just a mishmash of the day's events, anxiety dreams where my deepest fears are acted out, and prophetic dreams, which are the ones which carry a real message. I'll outline two such dreams here, which enabled me to make a couple of very big decisions:

I was having a real struggle with the information I'd uncovered and the seriousness of the situation. I had to make a decision as to whether to go conventional or alternative. I had grave doubts about conventional treatment and getting information about alternative treatment all seemed a bit 'underground'. I was having to sift the facts from amongst cranks and people out to financially exploit vulnerable cancer patients.

I asked, by writing in my diary, for a definition of conventional treatment. In the dream which followed, I found myself with my two elder brothers. One of them was in a wheelchair, and we took him to a huge public building where many other people were waiting. We approached a man on a desk, who was sitting beside a huge machine. He took my brothers' details and my brother died right on cue. He was then put through the machine and processed, as I and my other brother waited in a room in tears. I asked my brother how could he have just died? It didn't make sense that all those people were just waiting there to be processed, none of them questioning. At the end of the process we were handed my brother's remains in a box and we had to go back to the desk. The man on the desk was handing over to another who was a

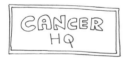

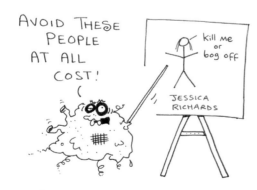

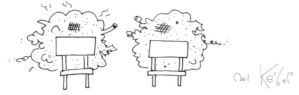

lot less serious. The first man reminded the second not to be too frivolous, as the people were facing a very traumatic situation. The second man ignored him, and continued to process the crowd one by one. Everyone just went along with it without question.

It seemed very clear to me that I'd dreamt of a 'Cancer Machine' in which we're all processed. We even tend to die when we're told we will.

I had another request to ask in my diary shortly afterwards. 'Show me the likely outcome if I choose Dr Andre Young-Snell and the alternative route' I wrote.

In the dream which followed this, I found myself and my partner Alan sitting at a consultant's desk. The consultant was at the far corner of the room, bent over the table looking through a microscope. As we sat down he looked up beaming and said, "I'll put you out of your misery, you're extremely healthy." I had my answer, and my decision! And it felt right.

A few weeks later I went to Dr Andre's clinic in Brighton to begin a three-week course of Vitamin C infusions where I really got to know and love this delightful man. As we walked past his desk into the adjoining room, there he was, in the far corner bent over the table mixing the Vitamin C with the saline ready for infusion, in exactly the position I'd seen him in my dream!

"Going within' is the taking of a journey in which the self leaves the mind and travels to the soul, where one's personal story does not exist. This allows you to come from a totally different space as you look at what is happening to you. You go to a different space so that you can come from a different space." Neal Donald Walsh - When Everything Changes, Change Everything.

I notice even now, a few weeks before I'm due to go back to the hospital for an appointment with Mr Kissin, I've started to have dreams about him and the hospital visit. So far, the dreams have all been along the same lines, Mr Kissin has his arm around my shoulder laughing and happy. This certainly takes some of the stress out of having the scan, examination and blood tests.

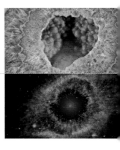

CHAPTER 6

 # Don't die, it's embarrassing!

Ten ways not to die

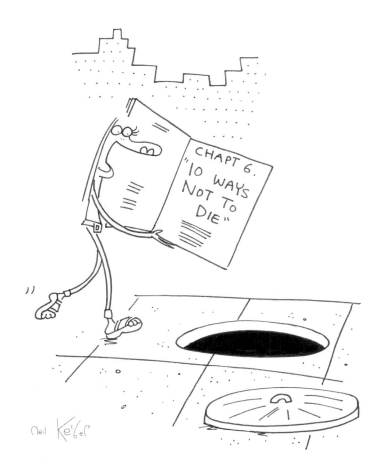

1. laugh

"There is nothing that can withstand the onslaught of laughter". Mark Twain

I don't feel a day has been lived fully unless I've laughed myself to tears at least once. It's not always possible of course but it can happen even in the direst situations. I know you will probably be thinking, "What the heck have I got to laugh about, I've been diagnosed with cancer?" What are you going to do then, cry about it all day? I know that, whatever treatment you choose, you will probably be with other people in the same boat for at least some of the time and it can lead to bit of 'gallows humour' but there are other ways to lighten the atmosphere and your load.

Try to hang out with cheerful people and those who make you laugh. Watch your favourite comedy shows or films. A friend of mine, Tim Hancock, gave me the full boxed set of 'Only Fools and Horses' as well as 'Hancock's Half Hour' and 'Dad's Army', all of which gave me a laugh. Being serious will not make cancer go away whereas it is a scientific fact that laughter strengthens our immune system. And our immune system is our most powerful ally to recovery.

BEFORE WE EMBARK UPON ANYTHING DRASTIC LIKE CHEMOTHERAPY, I'D LIKE TO TRY AN INTENSE COURSE OF TICKLING !

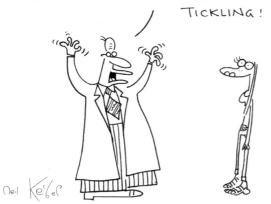

Neil Kerber

2. be enthusiastic

Be enthusiastic about something, anything. It may be a special plan for the future. It may be your family, your garden, or a car - whatever turns you on. I became enthusiastic about the idea of this book. It gave me something to think about that would provide a useful service for others in the same situation. I just thought, if I've got to have cancer, I'm darn well not going to have it for nothing! Just make sure it's something that really floats your boat and serves you in a way that makes you feel good about who you are. Don't worry about having the odd off day, we all have those. We can't be 'Pollyanna' all the time, that's not normal (those of you who know the story will remember that even she went 'off the boil' a bit after an accident) but do make the effort when you can.

3. individuate yourself

While you are having your chosen treatment, make sure you are treated as an individual and not just another cancer patient. This will empower you to take charge of your own treatment and will ensure that you are satisfied you are getting the right treatment for you at any given time and not just the 'one size fits all' treatment. This will also make it easier for you to ensure that things happen when they should and you don't slip through the net.

A friend of mine had anal cancer and was treated successfully. However, over recent years she'd noticed swollen lymph nodes in her neck and sore throats, amongst other symptoms. It was known that she also had a strong genetic predisposition to cancer and many of her female relatives had died prematurely due to it. The later symptoms were never investigated and nine years after her first diagnosis she called me to tell me that she now had cancer in her throat, tonsils and lymph nodes of her neck. I haven't included this to scare anyone, simply to illustrate that, although relatively rare, mistakes can and do happen. So I urge you to be vigilant in knowing what is happening, and persistent if you feel unsure about anything. You don't have to become an expert on cancer, but you can become an expert on yourself. It will help to make you feel empowered and in control of the situation and you may find you've been worrying for nothing.

4. remain present

This one is vital (see chapter 5 on mental attitude). Stay with the current facts of your situation and don't allow your mind to wander into 'What if?' or 'Why?' territory. Deal with today and what you know right now. Continue to make plans for your future but remain in the present when thinking about your health situation. Remaining present and fact-focussed will keep you positive and in control which is great for your state of mind and wellbeing.

5. question everything

Never, ever, go along with any treatment based purely on assumption or belief. Regardless of the treatment you choose, whether it's a particular type of drug or surgery or some wonder vitamin, ask what, why and how, until you are satisfied it's the best choice for you.

Again: You don't have to become an expert on everything, just become an expert on yourself. There's nothing wrong with going along with what most people do so long as you've thoroughly investigated what happens to most people and you feel OK about the possibility of that happening to you.

6. exercise

We all know we should exercise but do we really know why? The fitter your body, the healthier you are and the more likely it is that your immune system will be functioning well. Aerobic exercise, where you use your heart and lungs on a regular basis, will keep your system oxygenated which, in turn makes it a hostile environment to cancer cells. Keeping flexible helps to keep everything functioning in good working order. You are working here to support your immune system and wreck the cancer environment in your body. Cardiovascular exercise will also metabolise adrenalin from stress, which can be a major factor in any illness.

Treat your body with respect. Start off gradually. I use an analogy of a racehorse. If you had a priceless racehorse that was facing a major health issue, you wouldn't just let it lie around and you wouldn't force it into full training. You would bring in an expert to design a specific programme to help the animal regain its health and strength.

I have an exercise regime which suits me, but I urge you to contact a qualified practitioner who can evaluate you and design a program which suits your personal needs and preferences.

Don't think you suddenly have to develop the fitness of an Olympic athlete, if you've been a couch potato for most of your life, or if you have physical difficulties which affect your ability. Just aim to 'up your game' and get fitter than you were. You'll be amazed at how your body will respond. It's designed to be fit and active.

If you have surgery, you will no doubt be given exercises from your hospital which will help you to heal and keep you flexible. When diagnosed, I was already extremely fit so I continued with my usual regime which I've since added to. I continued to run about 3.5 miles on most days, and included stretching exercises. I still run up to 5 days per week, I use weights to build muscle tissue and strengthen bones and I jive dance every week - and more often if I can!.

7. avoid negative and stressful situations and people

This is crucial for your frame of mind. A negative frame of mind can be very draining on the body. (Refer to Chapter 5) Have you noticed how being around very negative people can leave you feeling very drained? Well, this is the last thing you need during your treatment and recovery from cancer.

We constantly find ourselves in situations which can be life negating. I always ask myself the question, 'is this worth dying for?' This is the only rule of thumb I feel is relevant.

There are, of course, many stressful situations which are completely out of our control, but don't think this means you have no chance, because there are things you can do to limit the effects of stress.

Within three years of my diagnosis, I lost both my parents, split up with my partner of eleven years and went to the wall financially! There were many other awful occurrences during this time but I've remained physically well, with normal blood tests throughout. 'Going within' by meditation, relaxation and visualisation can be a life saver. You go within or you go without! Combine this with a healthy lifestyle and keep company with cheerful strong people.

So, as you see, I'm still alive and well even with nightmares to live through. I've had to dig very deep but, the way I see it, we're all going to die at some point anyway so I intend to give this life a thorough run for its money before I'm done with it. At the end of the day, there is absolutely nothing to lose! So, don't let stress become an issue. Remember, it's not what life presents to you which defines you who you are, but who you choose to be in relation to it.

8. watch your thoughts and keep them positive

Relax. Use a relaxation CD or meditate, whatever suits you. It gives your mind a rest and discharges stress which avoids a build-up. Learn something new or become more expert in something you already know.

There's something very life affirming contained in the satisfaction of learning something new or developing expertise in a familiar pursuit. I got quite addicted to jive dancing, as it not only releases stress and helps keep you fit, but it's possible to become more and more competent which, to me is a joy. I simply love the feeling as it falls into place and I become less awkward.

I've also decided to learn a language. I get a real kick when the fog begins to lift and I occasionally know what's going on. The other piece of learning I'm committed to is to become IT literate. It would save time, create opportunities to do things differently and to expand on what I am doing, and it would open a whole new world of communication and information. At the moment, I'm thrilled if I've managed to order a few books online! I am determined to make the whole thing less of a mystery, and even though it's not my strength, I want at least to be able to recognise competence in others when I need to. Learning something new helps you remain present.

9. *eat well, play well, sleep well*

Treat your body with respect. It needs time to recover. Make sure you get enough rest. I've known people proudly announce that they've never stopped working, no matter how ill they were feeling. I know it's good to carry on with normal life as far as possible but don't risk literally working yourself to death. No-one will thank you for it and there's really nothing to prove.

Take time out whenever possible, perhaps with children, family or friends. This can really help to bring back a feeling of normality. Eat an alkaline diet of whole foods and remember that alcohol is poisonous. (Refer to Chapter 4 on Things not to eat and drink). The only symptom I felt before I was diagnosed was an extreme exhaustion which I couldn't sleep off. One of the secretaries where I work at Harley Street, described me as looking as though I'd just got off a long haul flight, and this was in the morning before I'd even started work! When I started my treatment plan, I allowed myself as much sleep as I needed. Normally I'm an early riser and have always found it impossible to have a lie in, or to return to sleep after waking in the morning. What I noticed was that, at first, I was sleeping twelve hours or more straight through. After a short time, I was waking up earlier and feeling like I'd actually had some sleep! This continued until I was back to my normal early rising habits and feeling refreshed. This was a good sign to me that my body was returning to normal.

Avoid environmental toxins as these put pressure on your immune system. Remove toxic cleaners and personal care products which contain chemicals as far as possible. There is much evidence to suggest that a constant bombardment of chemicals in our daily cleaning and toiletry products can affect our health. We do have the power to make a difference here and one which will also have a positive effect on the environment. Changing your cleaning products can also save you a fortune. I use distilled white vinegar and bicarbonate of soda for cleaning, using the vinegar as a fabric softener and as a rinse aid in the dishwasher. I also make my own spray polish from white vinegar and boiled linseed oil, but I mainly use Kangen Water for all kinds of cleaning.

10. *be thankful*

What you appreciate, appreciates. I'm not being patronising here. Gratitude actually affects your body chemistry just as other emotions such as love, hate, and fear do. It's simply a biological fact. No matter what situation we're in, there's still something to be found in the simple things like seeing the start of another new day, the love of family and friends, bulbs coming up in the spring. I love the feeling of being physically aware whilst I'm running or dancing and can feel my heart and lungs working and the blood coursing through my veins. I like to run outside in the open where I can smell the earth and sense the changes in the seasons. There is something very life affirming about being in touch with nature and you don't have to run through it, walking or even shuffling or sitting in it will do.

Whilst we are physical beings, we have the capacity to communicate and interact with others. I remember a dream where I fell from a balcony and smashed my body. As others gathered around my lifeless body I became aware of the impossibility of telling them that I was still there, but just out of my body. Even the most psychic of them was barely aware of my presence. I felt sad and frustrated that I had been so careless as to break my body. It seemed far more of a spiritual experience to be in it and interacting on a physical level.

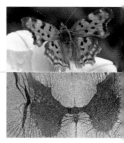
butterfly

spinal column cross section

CHAPTER 7

 # I don't know what to say to someone with cancer.

Ten things not to say to cancer patients, and how not to put your foot in it

Firstly, there are no right or wrong things to say, as everyone is different. I've just included things which I found unhelpful and the things most often mentioned by others who were dealing with cancer. Before I begin, I would like to make it clear that I am profoundly grateful to anyone who tried to help, in whatever way they tried, even if they did fall into some of these traps! I'd said some of these things myself, until I found myself on the other side of the fence.

People will say the strangest things but it's important to remember that they really don't mean anything by it. They just don't know what to say. I think it's really important to try to treat people with kindness and compassion even though you're the one with cancer. However their comments come across, they invariably have a noble origin and if someone feels they've upset you they can be quite devastated by it. Can you imagine, they've not only upset someone they care about but they've upset someone with cancer! It's a funny thing, when you have cancer you often have to take more care of other people's feelings than ever.

Anyway, here are my top ten things not to say to cancer patients, based on my experience:

1. "Ooh, I knew someone who had that and it spread everywhere."

Believe it or not, people actually say stuff like this. They don't mean anything by it, some people simply panic and say the first thing that comes into their mind because they don't know what to say or how to react. They spill it out before they've had a chance to think.

I remember when I'd just told a friend of mine that I'd been diagnosed with breast cancer and

would be having a lymph node biopsy the following week. He replied, "That's what happened to a friend of mine, he had cancer of the lymph. He suffered so much, but they couldn't save him and he died about a year later." I blinked a couple of times and told him that we all have our cancer anecdotes, even me, but they're never helpful and stories like that are particularly unhelpful. He got the message.

We all know what can happen if you have cancer, and although it's not a good idea to lie to people it's worth bearing in mind that there are some things they really don't need reminding of. My father said one of the most helpful things to me. Just after I told him I was being treated for cancer and had decided against chemotherapy and other conventional treatments, he followed me into the kitchen and said "Have you told me everything?" I assured him that he knew as much as I did, and that I would never leave him unprepared. Then he said, "That's good enough for me and whatever treatment you choose, I know you'll make the right decisions for yourself because you're a winner." He never did question my choices and always showed complete confidence in my ability to make sound judgements (regardless of what he must have been feeling). Another thing I found helpful was when a friend simply said to me, "It's just another illness."

If you're in a group situation, please treat a cancer patient the same as everyone else. I've been in groups, where someone would join us, and do the usual jovial greetings with everyone, and then turn to me and adopt a sympathetic, pitying look, and say 'and how are you?' We're not different, and we're not dead, so please don't change towards us, or treat us differently.

2. "My life's a mess, my house was struck by lightning, I lost my job, my dog got run over, cost me three thousand pounds at the vet and he died anyway, but that's nothing compared to what you're going through."

I had to laugh to myself when I was re-reading this during editing, as these were some of the things which actually happened to me. My two cats died at fourteen and fifteen years and the third who decided to move in with me got hit in the face by a car (but fortunately survived after some expensive jaw wiring). My neighbour's house suffered a direct lightning strike which blew everything electrical from the walls in my house and paying privately for treatment has almost sent me to the wall financially! However, it really doesn't help to think that everyone believes cancer is far worse than anything else that can possibly happen to anyone.

Now, I would laugh and say, "I'll be so pleased when I'm no longer the criteria for a crap life. What you've described sounds far worse than my life."

To be honest, apart from the beginning, and once I'd got used to the idea, (and you do) and I'd decided on my treatment plan, it was certainly no picnic but I was never unwell. My alternative treatments were quite benign, so I was just stressed out and poor! It really helps not to have people walking around on eggshells. I, and others I've spoken to, simply crave normal mundane things and conversations. Please try not to remind us how grim or frightening you think our situation is.

3. "You're so brave."

No I'm not, it's not a lifestyle choice, I wasn't asked if I could handle cancer and bravely replied 'yes', I simply got told I had it and there was no option. There's nothing brave in getting diagnosed with cancer then having to deal with it.

I remember visiting a friend in hospital after her third major cancer surgery and it was borderline as to whether she would have to lose her bladder. At this point, because of the nature of her surgery she was unable to eat normally and had just sucked ice cubes for the previous two weeks. When we were alone, she looked at me and said, "To be honest, I really don't think I could go through all this again," There was a second's silence before we both burst out laughing with the same thought. It's not as though there would be a choice! Regardless of whether we think we can go through it or not, we have to.

You may think that you couldn't handle it but, like us, you would because there's no choice.

It almost feels patronising to be told we're brave, because bravery doesn't come into it for most of us. On the other hand, when I'd decided to go the completely alternative treatment route, my friend Joanna said, "I'm right behind you because you're doing this for all of us. We don't know who'll be next and we need people like you to show there may be a different way."

4. "This may help you on your cancer journey"

I'm sure I'm not the only person to find this a bit of a cliché and even a bit patronising.

To me it was far from a 'journey' and for most it's more like a trip to hell. I remember one particularly stressful and shocking discussion with surgeons where they'd decided I should have a mastectomy rather than a lumpectomy and I'd responded that the news was getting worse at every meeting. The nurse said, "Well it's not an exact science, it's more of a 'journey' really." I did not find this at all comforting. It felt more like running the gauntlet than anything else. If anyone else mentions the word 'journey' I simply answer that everyone says that, but I can assure you it doesn't feel like a journey from this side of it.

Speaking from the heart is so much more meaningful than resorting to clichés. When I stayed with Alan's' mother Sheila, I was having a particularly challenging time, dealing with all the treatment and lifestyle changes as well as the uncertainty about the future. Sitting at the dining table one day, she said, "This is one of those times in your life that you just have to live through." That really summed it up and put it into perspective. Truly, all things must pass.

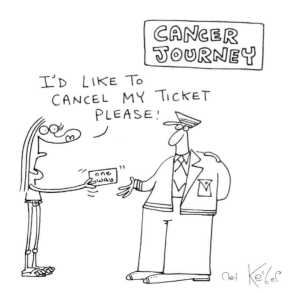

5. "I'm sure you'll win your battle with cancer."

In the first place, you don't know whether someone will survive or not and it really doesn't help to have one person after another making the same pointless comment. As my consultant said, only time will tell if you will survive or succumb, and this is it, only time will tell, absolutely nothing and no one else can. Secondly, I know it's fashionable to refer to it being a 'battle' but I didn't want to feel I was in a "battle". I know that many who choose a conventional route find it's a long, hard slog and few feel like warriors! And what does it say about those who don't make it? They didn't battle hard enough? They didn't put up a big enough fight?

I didn't catch cancer, it didn't just fly through my window, it was growing in my body, and if I was to fight or do battle with it, I would be fighting and doing battle with myself. Instead of declaring war on, and fighting with my own body, I concentrated on providing my body with everything it needed to be well. This included supporting my immune system, the only real expert on dealing with cancer, or any other diseases. At the same time, my treatment was specially designed to wreck the cancer environment within my body without wrecking me.

Along with this, is the importance of being careful not to see death as a failure. We're all going to die at some point, it's inevitable and unavoidable. When someone dies, it doesn't mean they've failed especially when they've done everything within their power to recover. I've known several people who've died years after they were given just weeks or months to live, and have lived normal and fulfilling lives in the meantime. Others choose their own route and have a normal family life for the year or so they have left. Some fulfil a special goal whilst others create something of great value to others. Some consciously choose to take the opportunity that disease gives them to leave their life on their own terms. Life is sweet but it's sweet in different ways to different people and we should understand and respect that, as well as understanding those who succumb after a heroic effort to stay alive. You can rest assured they'd have gone a lot sooner had they not made the effort. There is no failure here.

I know some people consider my story a success, because I'm alive and well. I can tell you, this is not how I define success for myself. As I've said before, success, for me, is living or dying on my own terms.

6.   "Oh, I'm sorry to hear that, well . . . keep in touch and let me know how you're doing."

When you are diagnosed, you're overwhelmed with information, appointments, rearranging life, considering death, and asking and answering questions. You don't need the extra commitment of keeping people updated. Real friends keep in touch and help where they can. People who ask more of you may want to appear caring and concerned but probably can't be bothered to make the effort themselves. The couple of people who said it to me didn't get any calls from me, and they never bothered to call me!

7.   "Are you cured yet?"

People are even more inclined to say this if you take an alternative route. When someone has conventional treatment, everyone expects it to be a long-term process and we know it can be two or three years before someone is given the 'all clear'. It's even worse for celebrities and others in the media spotlight. As soon as he or she has announced the end of chemotherapy or surgery, they're proclaimed as cured. After a cancer diagnosis, we are never really free of it, it is always in the background of our life. I found that because I'd chosen a different approach, everyone seemed to expect some miracle cure in a matter of weeks. Well, there is no miracle cure: we don't have a cure at all for cancer. I found it most unhelpful to be put under this pressure. Everyone seemed to expect it to be over in a few short weeks, with the inference that, if I wasn't 'cured', then my treatment obviously wasn't working.

I would like to add a note here about my experience in choosing an alternative route of treatment. I believe I received less sympathy and understanding than that afforded to other cancer patients. Because I looked well, then I couldn't be 'that' ill. I was 'lucky' because I didn't 'have' to have chemotherapy, and so on. I felt I had to hide my treatment in front of other patients as though it was a secret crime. I was even compared on more than one occasion to more well-known cancer patients with comments like, "Well, hers was really serious" , with the inference that mine wasn't.

Many people I've spoken to have been upset by comments such as "Oh you look well", especially to those who've received a bleak prognosis. It is usually said with a note of surprise. I would often respond with, "well I'm not dead yet if that's what you mean." I also understand that in my case, I did look well for most of the time because of my benign treatment and high level of fitness. Most people don't realise it's often the treatments that make someone ill when they have cancer. Very often we hear in the media that, "oh so – and – so lost their hair because of their cancer."Well they didn't, they lost their hair because of the chemotherapy treatment!

The thing is, it's worrying when someone tries to convince you that you look well when you're seriously ill. If someone really is looking well and you know them well enough then fine, do say so, but otherwise it's best to say nothing. When I was first diagnosed and was facing chemotherapy and surgery, before I'd decided on the alternative route, I asked my friend Tim Hancock if he'd come to visit me and he replied, "Of course, I wouldn't miss out on an opportunity to mock the afflicted." This was the right response for me as it was normal for us to banter in this way.

8.   "You've got to keep positive."

I heard this on many occasions and found it very frustrating to have people keep repeating clichés to me as though it was the first time I was hearing them. I categorise this kind of advice as 'Bee in the drawers'. I'll explain. When I was about 22 years old, it was fashionable to wear essential oils as perfume. On this particular day, I was wearing a yellow flared skirt and a liberal splash of some sweet oil. I was waiting for a train in London, and I noticed a bee flying near me. I did my best to avoid it and got on the train. As we neared the next station I felt a burning sensation around my nether regions and realised the bee had got caught up in my skirt and had stung me. As the train pulled in, I leapt off, lifted my skirt up and dashed into the ladies where a cleaner was mopping the floor. I shouted, "quick! let me into a loo, I've got a bee in my drawers!" She replied in all seriousness, "ooh, you want to get that out!" Talk about stating the obvious!

It's pretty much a given that we have to keep positive, and unless you can follow your remark with some help as to how you might do that (see chapter 5) then it's better left unsaid. It feels a bit like when you're angry and someone tells you to 'calm down' or depressed and they tell you to 'cheer up' or worst of all, when you're perfectly happy and someone keeps telling you to 'smile'.

9.   "How is your cancer?"

Health professionals can be particularly prone to this but so can friends and family. The issue here is that psychologically, once we accept something as 'mine' we begin to own it on an unconscious level and on this level, we tend to want to hang on to something we own. I always refer to it as the tumour or just 'cancer' which gives a bit of psychological distance and therefore enhances a mental attitude which can aid recovery. Try it for yourself. Think of something you really don't want and refer to it as yours and then refer to it as, 'it' or 'the' and feel the difference.

I had a phone call with a friend I hadn't heard from for a while. After a bit of catching up she suddenly asked, "and how is your cancer?' For a second I was lost for words and then I felt a slight surge of anger. I know she meant nothing by it, but it really felt like she was considering it as an entity in its own right. I felt as though I should give her its phone number to call! My pet cancer! I mean, would you really ask someone, "How is your heart disease?" or "how is your MS, obesity, diabetes, infertility?"

Asking whether you're still in pain is also difficult. When someone is suffering, (and people really can suffer during cancer treatments or in the late stages of the disease) it can make matters worse to constantly make them focus on the miserable and frightening symptoms of the disease or treatments. The medics need to ask these questions in order to ensure the person has the right medication to help them deal with it but, unless you are able to offer relief it's far kinder and more helpful to focus on something else if they are well enough to talk.

Please don't make a big deal of it, if the cancer patient has a headache. There were a couple of people who, if I'd mentioned having a headache, or similar, would respond with 'Oh My God! Are you alright? Do you feel OK?' This would make me feel a bit frustrated, as I'd explain that I simply had a headache, or backache or whatever it was, just the same as anyone else. I mean, for heaven's sake, even cancer patients get normal aches and pains.

I remember a male colleague mentioning that I seemed to be losing weight, and one of my female colleagues saying how great it was that a man could notice such a thing. I laughed, and informed her that it was no such thing, and that it was simply because he thought I was starting 'the big fade'.

10.   "Have you read 'Such and Such'?"

Book and website suggestions are very helpful and well-meant but when you're under the stress of a cancer diagnosis, especially in the early days, there's simply not time to go through the endless recommendations of reading matter. That's actually the reason I wrote this book, to give immediate access to the information you need, when you need it. It should at least get you started. I'm actually an avid reader but the situation is overwhelming enough without having a pile of books and websites to read through.

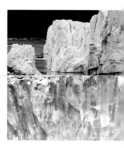

CHAPTER 8

Someone I care about has cancer, how can I help?

Ten practical ways to help someone after a cancer diagnosis.

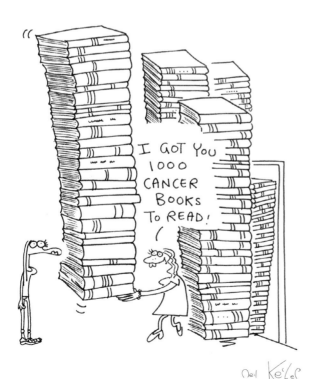

1. Gather information for them.

Check first if they would like you to do it, then, edit the information finding the relevant sections, so they don't have to trawl through the whole thing. I was bombarded with suggestions such as, "you must check out this website or that article". Under the circumstances, this felt totally overwhelming especially as I'm not someone who enjoys 'surfing the net'! I simply didn't have time to spend hours doing this, I'd just had a hand grenade thrown into my life and, at the time, I had no way of knowing how urgent it was or how fast I would have to act.

If you find a book, which may be helpful, don't just suggest that they read it. Believe me, I can't tell you how many books I was supposed to plough through to get to the odd relevant chapter.

My friend Marisa did a great thing; she read through the books herself and simply highlighted the parts that would be of interest to me. I've chosen to write this book in such a way that it's easy for you to go straight to the relevant chapter so you can access the information you need quickly.

2.   Be creative with your sympathy.

If you hear someone close to you has cancer I know how helpless it can make you feel. You just want to do something. Please think twice before you send flowers. If you want to send a card, try to make it positive. No-one wants to be reminded of how grim and serious their situation is. Flowers are questionable. Personally, I felt my lounge looked a bit like a funeral parlour and was a reminder of how bad my situation was as far as my friends were concerned.

One lady who was at Dr Andre's clinic at the same time as I was, told me that instead of buying flowers, her friends had clubbed together to replace her toiletries and cosmetics with ones made with natural ingredients. This is such a great idea as, no matter what treatment you choose, personal and household products which are free from chemicals can be a great asset. Environmental chemicals put an extra strain on your immune system at a time it needs all the help it can get.

So, why not think about natural cosmetics and cleaning products?

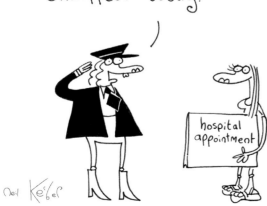

3.   Help with travel.

When first diagnosed, there can be a lot of travelling involved to various hospital and clinic appointments as well as complementary practitioners. It can be a great help to have a driver, either for the person concerned or so that their spouse or family member can have a day off.

You won't always know what's best but most people, when asked, will tell you that they can manage. Sometimes it's easier for them if you just say what time you'll be there and suggest going for a bit of lunch or a cup of tea afterwards, depending on time available and how they're feeling.

I remember when I told a small group of close friends and asked them not to start giving me advice or anecdotes as I was getting a bit overwhelmed. Luckily my friend Marisa ignored it and got some information for me, which was seriously helpful as well as making arrangements for me to stay at her house prior to surgery. She didn't ask, she just made the arrangements, fed me and drove me to the hospital.

4.   Be a satellite person.

If you are close, offer to be the go-between who relays latest information to friends and relatives who know about the situation. This will save them from having to think and talk about cancer virtually non-stop. As I mentioned in a previous chapter, I had what I call 'satellite' people in various aspects of my life who relayed news and information in those areas. When my mother died, Alan took on the job of telling my friends and neighbours and letting them know that I would prefer them not to send sympathy cards or flowers as I would find it too distressing to have these reminders around me.

Please remember however, that unless you are asked to give information to someone else, or to discuss anything with a third party, don't.

5.   Help with the mundane.

If the person has children or elderly parents to care for, you can help out, perhaps by taking the children out for the day or taking them to and from school and other activities. You can also help take care of older parents and maybe bring them for a visit. I can't stress enough how important it is to help out with the everyday mundane things. The sort of things which need doing on a daily or weekly basis. A friend of mine had a team of friends who worked out a rota for household chores.

Keeping someone's house vacuumed or garden tidy can make a big difference to how they feel and don't forget about walking their dog or feeding other pets. The key here is to make it regular if you can, even if it's only once a month. Don't forget to keep someone's car going too if they're unable to drive it for prolonged periods.

The big gesture of help is always welcome but it's the everyday things that can really get on top of someone. You may also be able to help in your professional capacity, offering things like accounting, or hairdressing and so on.

6.   Personal care.

This is a delicate area but it can also be a very important one. Your friend or loved one may have trouble with personal care such as shaving, bathing, haircare, manicures and pedicures which are not only 'feel good' treatments but can have an impact on health and general wellbeing. I know when some men get ill and are either unable or just can't be bothered to shave , they can look and feel even worse, whereas being clean shaven in clean clothes with cut fingernails and toenails can make them feel and look a whole lot better.

When undergoing cancer treatment, it can seem like a never-ending road of unpleasant treatments and incremental bad news. It can make a real difference to experience pleasant physical contact. Depending on how well you know the person, consider at least a foot or hand massage, as it can be very soothing and greatly help with pain control and immune system support whilst avoiding areas where they may have had surgery or are experiencing discomfort. I remember during my mother's illness when massaging her arms and legs brought a great deal of peace and comfort to her.

7.   Help with a specialist diet.

If the person concerned is sticking to a special diet as part of their treatment it would be a great help to them if you could source ingredients for them and perhaps devise some recipes, and even prepare some meals. My friend Astrid loves to have people round to her house for food and drinks. She learned what she could about my diet and catered for me at these events where everything else just carried on as normal. This was a great help as I'd practically given up on going out to eat as it was just too complicated and I was fed up with explaining to everyone what I could and couldn't have. It was bad enough having to live with it without having to keep talking about it.

Remember, if someone is having conventional treatment, they may feel very tired and/or nauseous. If they're tired, help with preparing a nutritious meal could be very welcome, whereas if they're feeling or being sick, keeping them hydrated is more important than eating. Nobody can face eating when they feel sick.

8.   A bit of light relief, and some light diversions.

Catch a film, show, or other event, or maybe offer a day in the country or at the seaside. It doesn't have to be very elaborate or take very long. Between Christmas and the New Year of 2008 I had a Vitamin C infusion treatment with Dr Andre in Brighton and Astrid drove down with me. Whilst I was having the infusion she wrote up some recipes on my laptop as I dictated them and after the infusion we went down to the seafront and had a bit of lunch and a cup of tea followed by a look round some of the more unusual shops where I encouraged her to buy an outrageous pair of gold boots! It made driving all that way and having treatment so much more like a normal outing for us.

My friend Mary traced a lot of my family tree which was not only fascinating but gave me something else to think about and talk about, especially with my family. I also did an ancestral DNA test, which I found to be hugely interesting and surprising. It also gave me the chance to check out the cause of death for certain relatives. Interestingly, none I checked died from cancer!

9.   **Read aloud.**

Whatever treatment someone chooses, it can be a tiring process. It can be very relaxing to get involved in a work of fiction, one of the classics, articles from a favourite magazine or anything else for that matter which may be of interest and not necessarily to do with cancer. It can be a real gift to read for someone who is too tired to read for themselves. Talking Books are also great. Alan bought me a digital radio so that I could listen to plays and stories, and I carried that radio all around the house with me as well as in the garden. I still listen to the radio every day.

10.   **Teach them more about something of interest to them.**

During the initial three weeks at Dr Andre's clinic I stayed with Alan's mother Sheila. Sheila is an experienced and avid knitter and I thought that knitting was something I could do whilst chatting or watching the TV as well as being productive, and I was often too tired to read. We went into town to buy a pattern and some wool and I found it to be a wonderful distraction especially during the dark, winter months. I learned a lot about the subject - and I had a few dodgy jumpers at the end of it!

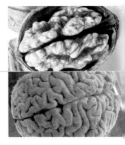

CHAPTER 9

 # What are the main points again?

A ten point checklist

Here's a checklist for you, so you can re-cap and cover all your bases quickly and think logically and practically about your situation.

1. diagnosis

Get a diagnosis that you understand even if it means getting a second, third and fourth opinion. I emphasise that this means a diagnosis that you understand, rather than the diagnosis you would prefer. Until you have a definitive diagnosis (as far as possible) you cannot begin to make a plan.

2. paperwork

It is absolutely vital at all times that you keep proper track of your paperwork. Make sure you get copies of everything concerning your situation and keep it in a file. This will enable you to keep track of everything that's going on as well as providing all your health care practitioners with the same up-to-date information.

AND JUST TO CONFUSE YOU EVEN MORE, HERE'S YOUR DIAGNOSIS IN ANCIENT EGYPTIAN HIEROGLYPHIC SCRIPT!

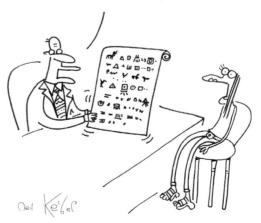

Neil Keibel

3. remain present

This is probably the most important mental element at this point. It's very difficult to keep positive, and you'll probably want to punch people who keep telling you to do it, but you can force yourself to remain present and just deal with the facts that you have right now. This is actually a way to be positive. Being positive can be a proactive thing rather an abstract, intangible concept.

4. water

Get the cleanest supply of water you can and work your way up to drinking 2 litres per day. Make sure that your water supply is as alkaline as possible. Most bottled water is acidic, whereas tap water can be either acidic or alkaline depending on the area you live, and needs a filter to remove chemicals and hormones. If you choose something like Kangen Water, it can be adjusted during chemotherapy or radiation treatments as it's a strong anti-oxidant and, as with all anti-oxidants, it can negate certain treatments which rely on oxidation for their efficacy. However, it can be extremely beneficial between treatments and at other times.

5. diet

Get the appropriate food and drink into your house. Whatever your diagnosis, eating an alkaline diet whilst tending to your other nutritional requirements can greatly assist in your recovery, whatever treatments you choose. This is something you can take care of immediately but do seek a qualified nutritionist who can advise you on a tailor-made regime appropriate for your own particular situation.

6. chemicals

Remove chemicals from your environment. This includes any household and personal products which contain potentially harmful chemicals. Replace them with natural products as far as possible.

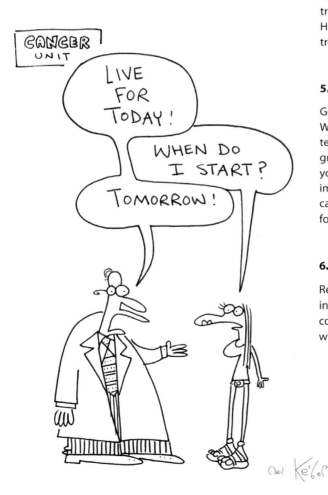

7. juicer

Invest in a juicer. You can buy them very cheaply these days and it doesn't matter much which one you choose to get you started. It's an easy way to get the vitamins and minerals you need especially if you've lost your appetite.

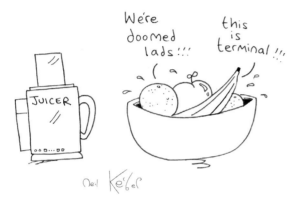

8. choose your hospital or clinic

Investigate which hospital and/or clinic would best serve you. This isn't just a practical issue of accessibility or facilities, but also an emotional one. Do you feel relatively safe and comfortable there and do you have confidence in those treating you there?

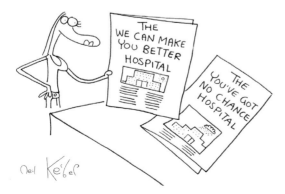

9. relaxation

Make time for relaxation. Just fifteen minutes a day will do to start but you must make sure it's dedicated time, and not to be relinquished except in a dire emergency. You cannot multi- task during this time. Go to a quiet place where you feel safe, Meditation is ideal, or put on some soft music or open the window and listen to the sounds of nature, or get lost in a recording of a favourite novel or poem. You are also welcome to the free relaxation download available from my website www.jessicarichards.co.uk Do whatever feels right for you.

10. team members

Begin to think about your team members and whether they are your choice, or if you've just accepted health professionals who've been allocated to you. Begin with one person you can trust and rely on and remember, it's ultimately *your* choice who's in your team.

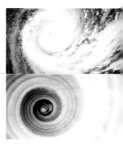
CHAPTER 10

Questions we should all be asking

1. **The National Health Service is funded by taxpayers, so why does it offer only one service for cancer and other diseases?**

With more and more people choosing an integrated approach to health care which includes complementary or alternative treatments, why do health care providers not offer or provide an integrated treatment approach?

We all fund the NHS and many pay additionally for private insurance, yet if the treatment programme offered does not serve us, we have to self-fund an alternative. Some conventional treatments have a very poor track record yet are still provided whilst other popular alternative or complimentary treatments are ignored or, if provided are very much hit-and-miss. Why do people like me and others who choose an alternative or integrated pathway of care have to resort to loans or re-mortgages to pay for it?

2. **Why, when it is generally accepted that diet and nutrition has a critical impact on our health and wellbeing, is it almost completely ignored by medical science when it comes to cancer and most other diseases?**

There is very little dietary advice available within the NHS and what little there is, is inconsistent and very much 'luck of the draw'. Isn't it about time that health care includes diet and nutritional advice as part of a basic package? I know that not everyone will follow the advice, but surely we have a right to the information in order to make the choice.

3. **Why aren't children educated in diet, nutrition and other health and wellbeing issues such as social awareness and social skills which would enhance their overall psychological, emotional and physical wellbeing?**

4. **Why is genuinely healthy food so difficult and expensive to acquire whilst processed food is piled floor-to-ceiling in most food retail establishments?**

5. Why don't some hospitals offer tumour marker blood tests to NHS patients?

They are available for private patients. This again seems to be a bit of a lottery. There is much debate and opinion about the value of tumour markers and I know that a blood test cannot tell you if you have cancer but regular tests for tumour markers would indicate a change earlier than finding a lump or having it show up on a mammogram or other scan.

Here is what I believe is the bottom line on this: I was a patient at a major cancer hospital and I asked this question: If I go through with all the treatment recommended, how will I know I am clear, and if I stay clear? I was told that I would be given mammograms to check if the cancer had recurred, and I was told that the NHS doesn't do blood tests. When I enquired why, I was told they had very little value. At the same time, the wife of a friend of mine was being treated for breast cancer at the same hospital under the same consultant and was having regular blood tests. The difference between us? She was a private patient and I was an NHS patient. So, what's the story? Either there is some value to having regular tumour marker blood tests and some hospitals withhold these from NHS patients to save money or the private health insurers are being ripped off!

6. Should we continue with a 'kill or cure' attitude towards cancer when it's possible that in many cases it can be controlled, as in other metabolic diseases such as diabetes?

7. Why is exercise advocated for disease prevention, but excluded in the treatment?

There is much evidence to suggest that exercise can greatly assist in the recovery from disease, not least because of the psychological effect of being able 'to do something' to help oneself.

8. Every city in the western world has at least one huge building dedicated to disease management (hospitals). Why don't we have any public centres dedicated to health and wellness management?

Surely it would make sense to use available funds to create public centres where people can learn and have access to everything they need to lead a healthier and more active life. This would free up medical staff and resources. Although we obviously need hospitals, it seems insane to me that we have access to 'health care' only when we're already in big trouble.

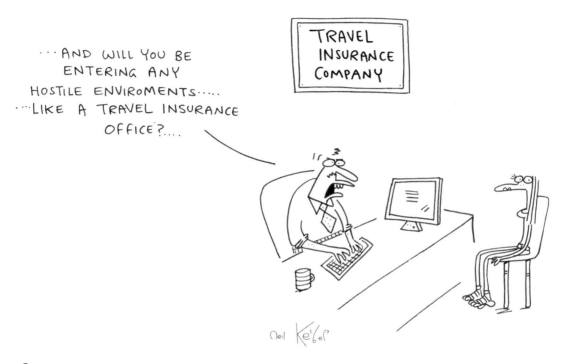

...AND WILL YOU BE ENTERING ANY HOSTILE ENVIROMENTS..... ...LIKE A TRAVEL INSURANCE OFFICE?....

TRAVEL INSURANCE COMPANY

9. **Why are travel insurance companies allowed to exclude cancer treatments when the customer didn't have cancer at the time of taking on the insurance?**

Just over a year after I'd been diagnosed, we were taking a short trip abroad. I called the travel insurance company to let them know of the diagnosis. The only reason for doing this was to make sure that if I did need the insurance because of accident or other illness, it wouldn't be invalidated because I hadn't disclosed new circumstances. I was told that cancer treatments would now be excluded from my insurance policy. They'd been happy to take my money for years but were then able to exclude something I might need it for. This needs to change. You wouldn't expect your car insurance company to exclude accidents on the day you report one would you?

10. **With little or no evidence to prove that we will be 'safer' especially given the track record of some pharmaceutical drugs, why are we being deprived of our right to choose our own pathway of care?**

By 2012 we will no longer be able to take responsibility for our own health in the way that I have, as legislation means we will be unable to buy high doses of certain herbs, vitamins and minerals. This is apparently for our own safety. Retailers and products will have to be licensed, and only those products in use for 15 years and over will be eligible for a licence.

Apparently, in ancient China, physicians received payment when the patient became well. What would happen if we applied this interesting concept to our present healthcare systems as well as to the producers of vitamins, drugs and herbs?

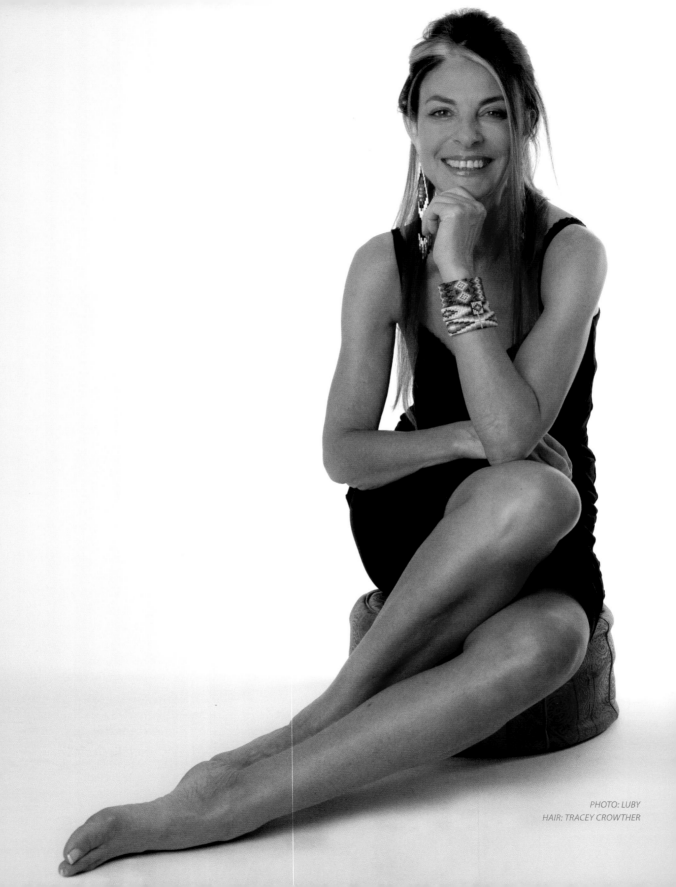

PHOTO: LUBY
HAIR: TRACEY CROWTHER

Afterword

Well, I'm still here and have still had no medical treatment. So whatever your situation, know that anything is possible and you have ultimate control over what happens to you.

Courage, determination and a strong mental attitude can all be learned.

Interviews with members of my team

I've interviewed some key members of my team, to give them a voice, and to ask on behalf of you, the reader, some more questions based on their expert knowledge and experience.

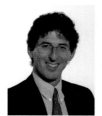

Mr Mark W Kissin
MA MB MChir FRCS

*Consultant Breast
and Melanoma Surgeon*

Mr Kissin is a specialist in breast cancer, and his comments refer specifically to this aspect of the disease.

Q: **In your experience and opinion, are there any commonalities in those who survive cancer either in character, age or physical characteristics?**

A: Although there's not a lot of scientific work to support it, it's my impression that a positive approach from a psychological point of view seems to be beneficial in terms of people who are very negative seem to have negative outcomes. In terms of age, age is no barrier to cancer or type of cancer but, some younger women tend to have more aggressive forms of cancer. On the other hand, they are better able to withstand more complex treatments because they are naturally younger, whereas people who have other medical conditions will be more at risk from complications of the treatments at a greater frequency. So, yes, age, type of person and general fitness can interface with things. We certainly know for instance that people who have high body mass index (obesity) have a worse outcome in hormone-related breast cancer.

Q: **Have you noticed any changes in patients' attitudes and choices of treatments since you've been in practice?**

A: Yes, I think that's because of the amount of information patients receive, from the media, from their general practitioner and from the breast care teams. Also, the breast care teams' better attitude and understanding on issues of communication and choice. So, plenty of studies show that where a choice is offered, psychological outcome is improved and there's a possibility that the cancer outcome is also improved, so sharing decisions with patients is usually of benefit. But, at the same time, you have to draw the line somewhere and not take control. Rather try and steer patients away from the wrong decisions and encourage them towards the right conditions.

Q: **Have your beliefs and attitudes changed since you started and if so how?**

A: When I first started as a consultant, twenty years ago, I had this slightly distorted opinion that I would be able to cure everybody and for the first two years I was absolutely right, nobody got a recurrence. Then everybody said to me, wait until two years are up, and of course the recurrences started, and that was a very sobering time. Looking at all the treatments we have at our disposal, you can see that maybe through slashing, burning and poisoning we can improve outcomes by ten, maybe fifteen percent across the board but that still means that we can't cure everybody and it still means that surgery alone would actually be curing the majority of patients with breast cancer.

The other thing that's happened in my working lifetime is the introduction and perseverance of breast screening, and in my opinion that's been a huge advance and much undermined by certain critics in the press. The outcome of screen-detected cancer in our region at the moment, over five years is 98.8%, you can hardly do better than that.

Q: **What do you feel is the future of cancer diagnosis and care?**

A: I think in terms of surgical procedures, and largely the other things seem to follow, we might be able to achieve more by doing less. But that doesn't mean to say that it's less complicated. So there are fewer mastectomies than there used to be and fewer wholesale lymph node removals than there used to be. Technology has improved to the extent that we can probe the genetics of cancer and design treatments very specifically for patients.

I think that individualised treatment will become the future as well as short-stay surgical care. Take for instance, the drug Herceptin. Why is it given for a year? Well, it's because one year was compared against two years and the result was the same. I suspect you would be able to give it for a much shorter space of time which would be more cost-effective. On the other hand, other treatments, such as hormonal blockade, might need to be given for a longer amount of time.

Q: **What about prevention?**

A: There was a recent article in Lancet Oncology which said we need to be concentrating on prevention. There are a variety of drugs which can prevent breast cancer. We know that Tamoxifen blocks oestrogen, but at a cost in terms of side effects, and you only need one bad side effect to cancel out the prevention aspect. The problem is that it's good at preventing 'good disease' and not good at preventing 'bad disease', so that's another side of the coin. Certainly one worries about the high body mass index you see walking around the high street, that is a definite risk factor, and the increased levels of alcohol consumption in younger women is of concern, as well as, to some extent, smoking.

There are plenty of things people can do, but remember we have an improved outcome in survivability in breast cancer and people are living longer across the board.

Q: **What do you know about the causes of cancer?**

A: Not as much as one might think. We can see a variety of things that tilt the odds against you. For instance, not having children at a young age and not breast feeding. Having periods that go on for a long time after fifty or start a long time before fourteen. Excessive amounts of HRT, excessive use of the oral contraceptive pill, smoking, drinking, being overweight, having a family history of breast cancer. Essentially, there's a lot we don't know and potentially a lot of cancer promoting agents in the food chain and water supply that contribute because cancer is a multi-step process. It's not going to be one thing that causes it.

Q: **Do you believe it's possible to treat cancer as a survivable metabolic disease such as diabetes, and manage it using it diet and lifestyle changes, rather than taking the 'kill or cure' approach most commonly applied in cancer treatment today?**

A: Truly, I have no idea and that's because we treat it in the usual way and we're not in the habit of not treating it. Anecdotally, some patients treating it in the 'not usual' way will do well, better than you might have anticipated whilst others perish in the way that you would suppose. So we don't know what the new natural history of the disease is and how it might be influenced. But we can't say that some of our treatments don't do harm because they do. However, on average the harm is easily outplayed by the good it can do.

Q: What advice would you give someone on receiving a cancer diagnosis?

A: I think number one, don't panic. Number two, you must feel confident and happy with your care team and if you're not, you must seek another care team. Also don't believe everything that is said and written about breast cancer because not all of it is true. Your cancer is not the same as someone else's and you can't extrapolate from one patient to another.

Q: What advice would you give new cancer consultants?

A: Be committed, don't ever lose the need to cross the Ts and dot the I's. You have to be anally retentive to be a good clinician, you must never let anything escape, and you can't delegate as much as you might want to because you can't assume everybody is as enthusiastic as you might be yourself. Also, remember that the patient knows more about their body than you do.

Q: What do you feel about supporting patients in their choices of treatment?

A: Fundamentally, it's very important, and it can be very difficult if the patient is given a conflict between their beliefs and your beliefs. It's even more important that they feel there is no conflict between the teams that are looking after her.

I have to say I'm a bit guilty about that because sometimes I try and make my beliefs override the beliefs of some of my colleagues which drives them completely bananas. Sometimes I may feel that they are not listening to what the patient is telling them.

Q: How do you feel about patients asking questions?

A: No problem, except if there are too many questions. Sometimes it's very helpful, it's very stimulating for a clinician to feel that the patient is on board and is doing their homework around the edge so they can know more and contribute, but sometimes that can be taken too far and you get some patients who seek opinion after opinion after opinion until they get the one that says exactly what they want it to say. At the same time, you've got to find an opinion that listens carefully as well as talks, so yes, questions are good.

Q: How do you feel when patients make you responsible and leave everything in your hands?

A: That's OK. It's the old maternalistic model of, "you know best Doc, do what you've got to do". It's not the right approach for many people in the modern world, but it's still the way that some patients want to go. You can spot this very quickly and when you spot it, there's no point in going into a deep discussion about the meaning of life. You just want to get on and deal with it and accept that it's up to you and the breast care nurses to identify these people and not try and overload them with communication when communication is clearly not required.

Q: How can patients best help you to help them?

A: I think the other side of the coin of me listening to them is for them to listen to me, so they need calmness and they need to have an understanding that breast cancer is not an acute illness. To some extent the media's attention to the disease is great because lots of money is coming into the research charities to enable us to do work and find things out, but the idea that it is a huge crisis when in fact, it must be developing over a period of months or maybe years sends the wrong signal to the patient. The impression is that something has to be done tomorrow, and that's not the biological truth.

To some extent, whilst the standards that have been set by various governments to have a certain treatment within a certain number of days is laudable because we don't want people to wait excessive times, the idea that you have to do something by a certain day otherwise the patient is compromised is totally false. Perhaps an example of that is, we are required to do the first surgical intervention within thirty one days after the decision to carry it out is made .The same is true of non invasive breast cancer as it is of invasive breast cancer, when clearly non-invasive breast cancer is, by definition, non-life threatening, and that doesn't make sense.

Q: **What would you like to see change in present day cancer diagnostics and treatments?**

A: Well it's changing all the time so there has been an evolution. In terms of surgical procedures we are in the era of euphemistically called onco-plastic surgery where we're trying to be destructive in a creative way to gain safety, gain knowledge, gain information yet render the patient as uninjured as possible. There's been a huge increase in performance and as such, we now have our own society of breast surgeons which I predict in the future will be a completely separate speciality from general surgery. Breast surgeons won't do 'on call', they concentrate on dealing with breast disease of all types, but nothing else.

Hormonal therapies are a little bit of a dead end. We've been able to block the oestrogen receptor, we can interfere with it, we can starve it, we can trick it. I don't see that there are many new drugs around the corner for that, there are just modifications for what we've got .Chemotherapy is coming on leaps and bounds and changing from intravenous drugs to oral drugs. The drugs for the future are going to be targeted, such as Herceptin but the problem is, those are very expensive to develop and therefore healthcare delivery becomes an issue. So shorter, sharper bursts of expensive drugs may be the thing for the future .

In terms of teams, better team working is being hugely beneficial and I think better use of people's time. As a surgeon, I like to operate and there's no point in my seeing hundreds of women who don't actually have anything wrong with them. It's much better that somebody who's a diagnostician can sift through these and find those who need my services rather than me having to do that.

Q: **What made you agree to monitor Jessica Richards?**

A: A sense of fairness, in that she was seeking to go down a different route from the one the satnav normally shows but the satnav's not always right in getting you where you need to be.

Q: **Would you like to add to the above?**

A: No, except to say that it's been a privilege and a pleasure to look after her.

Interview April 2011

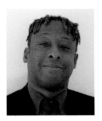

Dr Andre Young-Snell
MBBS

Dr Andre Young-Snell MBBS (Guys Hospital 1988) worked for many years in hospitals specializing in Parkinsons disease and Elderly Medicine. He led A&E emergency teams co-ordinating and designing patient treatments, and teaching junior doctors. He specialised in hospital medicine for 15 years, where he gained a great deal of experience treating cancer patients. He has been seeing patients at his Vision of Hope Clinic in Brighton since 2002

Outside Medicine he is very keen on music and is a songwriter in a band that has frequent shows around the country. As he says, 'The band has an ethos of inspiring people not to be apathetic and to do the most with their lives.' You can find him on www. Shootthedead.co.uk

Q: **You spent 20 years in the NHS, What caused or inspired you to set up an alternative health practice?**

A: I'm somebody who looks after my own health and I'm very keen to do the same for patients. The thing that really started me off was meeting someone called Tony Robbins, a motivational life coach. I went to see him about ten years ago and one of the things he was talking about , as well as doing the best to look after yourself ,was diet. We spent a day going through that and there were quite a few changes I realised I needed to make. I was a meat eater as well as eating all kinds of rubbish but this aspect of the course really changed me.

I came back to the hospital where I was working and a lot of patients were interested in what I was doing. During this time I was introduced to someone called Phillip Day who suggested that what I was doing on a small scale in the hospital, I could do on a much bigger scale with patients and the general public. So that was how I began to think about the sort of clinic I have now.

Q: **What, in your experience, is the most common factor in patients who survive?**

A: The most common factor is mental attitude, as in how that patient is mentally geared. We have audits every year, and it always comes up that patients who are very forthright, have goals and know what they want, tend to do very well whereas patients who are less sure about what to do and aren't mentally focussed, tend to do less well. What I mean by mentally focussed is having one or two clear goals that they are determined to make happen.

In addition, people who don't spend all of their time thinking about cancer do better, and those who, without necessarily acting as if they haven't got it, are careful not to let it take up all of their time, so they are busy doing other things and therefore putting their mental focus elsewhere.

Another interesting thing we've found is patients who have a strong spiritual or religious belief tend to do better than those who don't. This is not to say that you won't do well if you don't have a spiritual belief, just that generally speaking, those who do, tend to do slightly better.

It seems the common factor here is the F word as in Faith, a very important word. Those who have faith do well regardless of where that faith originates in terms of the type of spiritual or religious belief.

Q: **How can patients best help themselves?**

A: Patients can best help themselves firstly by relaxing. That may sound odd under the circumstances but it's important not to panic. A lot of patients, when told, tend to panic and think of the worst case scenario. That's understandable in the first instance but if they can relax and see this as a long term marathon rather than a sprint, that helps. So I would say, relaxing, not panicking and having goals are all very important. Mental attitude is a key thing.

Equally important and part of that mental attitude is having a sense of humour. Having fun and laughing is very important too. That might seem a bit odd, but it helps if someone is able to look at a bad experience and work out what the message is, what it is telling them and what opportunity lies within. A lot of people look at cancer as a terrible thing but the people who do well with me tend to look at the bigger picture and view it as a wake-up call.

Q: **Which protocols do you find most successful and does this vary with the type of cancer?**

A: On the whole, what I tend to use in my practice is a wide ranging approach. Once the patient has made their own informed decision to follow a complementary approach then I design protocols for them.

Cancer isn't one dimensional so there is no magic bullet. I find that using a wide range of protocols tends to work better for patients. If I were to pick one approach, then I would say the Vitamin C protocol is the thing we get best results from, whether it's intravenous or the new Lyposomal oral type which is also very good.

Another protocol I've found to be very effective (this is like trying to pick my favourite child here) is Ozone. We've been using that as well for a couple of years now and the overall results are even better, so I would say Vitamin C first and Ozone second.

Q: **Do you adapt protocols or advice according to the character of the individual?**

A: Yes 100%. We have to work with the patient. I like to work in a way which empowers people. What I mean by that is, a patient needs to feel important and special. Most patients don't feel this way when they come in, so it's very important to address it. Obviously, how you do that varies from patient to patient. Some people want you to be a buddy to them which means you can get very close to them and be quite informal, whereas other people have barriers so you can't do that and you have to interact in a different way. So you do have to gear

everything according to the patient's personality, yes.

Q: **Are you 'pro' an integrated system of treatment or are you completely alternative?**

A: I'm very much in favour of an integrated approach. In my dreams we have allopathic and complementary working much more closely together. In America there are many clinics which do that. There's a treatment called 'Insulin Potentiation Therapy' where, in a nutshell, patients are given insulin to lower their blood sugar followed by chemotherapy and Vitamin C. Many clinics in America as well as Mexico and Germany are providing this.

Unfortunately, we're not in that system so far in the UK. I would like to see that happen but I don't know whether I will see an integrated system of treatment available in this country in my lifetime. I do feel it's vitally important for treatment to be integrated.

Q: **What was your experience of cancer treatments before setting up your own practice?**

A: Having qualified at Guy's Hospital in 1988 I specialised in hospital medicine for many years before doing what I do now and had lots of experience giving chemotherapy and referring patients for radiotherapy and surgery. I also worked for 6 months at Guy's Hospital Breast Unit where breast cancer patients had surgery and received chemotherapy and radiotherapy, so during my time in the NHS I was working, not in specific cancer wards but in general wards where quite a few of the patients had cancer.

My personal experience in this situation was one of negativity, where a patient would be told he or she had cancer and there would be an aura of doom and gloom which is not the way I work.

Q: **What do you feel is the future of cancer treatments?**

A: I think the future of cancer treatments will be towards an integrated approach so basically, patients will have conventional and complementary therapies at the same hospital or clinic at the same time. I think there will be more focus on immune therapy and treatments to boost the patient's immune system. Also, there will be a lot more emphasis on prevention, by encouraging people to be fitter, looking after their diet, exercising, taking supplements and so on, as well as thinking differently about healthy lifestyle and goals, and looking after their emotional and mental health so that they won't be getting cancer in the first place.

Q: **You're in a band called 'Shoot The Dead', what's the story?**

A: The whole idea behind the name is not to take things literally at face value. Where I'm coming from medically, is to get people who are apathetic to be a lot more positive and a lot more goal-orientated with a lot more 'get up and go'. The band's name has similar connotations. What we're doing is getting people who may be lazy or apathetic to get off their backsides and to show passion and emotion and live a positive life. So, Shoot the Dead refers to being apathetic and uninvolved. That's where the name comes from and you can see that it fits in with my medical beliefs and general outlook on life. Apathy, lack of gratitude, lack of ambition and lack of spirituality are the scourge of our world and things that I fight with an absolute passion to discourage in others.

Q: **And the music of your band?**

A: It's kind of like a dance/rock crossover. It has very strong lyrics with a dance approach, so it's something to listen to and dance to.

Q: **Anything else you would like to add to the above?**

A: Yes. I don't have favourite patients as such but, if I did, they would be like Jessica because she embodies all of the characteristics common in those who have a positive outcome. When these patients come in they've thought about things and they know what they want. They tell me what they want and ask me how I can help them achieve that. Rather than coming in full of fear and saying things like, "Tell me what to do Doc."

So although ethically I can't help patients make decisions about whether they should have conventional or alternative treatment, I am here to help with the decisions they've made for themselves. These patients tend to have a forthright attitude and have extensively researched both sides so they have made informed decisions, know their own minds and are not easily swayed.

I would say that about one in 50 patients come in like this (others become like it over time) and to me, they are like gold dust because they ALWAYS do well and can have a very positive impact on other patients. I've seen patients who are virtually at death's door but pull themselves back when they have these other characteristics. This tends to happen when patients are faced with very few choices, so they are more able to make a definite decision and commit to it, whereas those who are given too many options and too many opinions at this point don't always do so well.

These patients tend to make decisions quickly, based on facts and change their minds slowly. They are not influenced by fear and they don't make cancer the centre of their thoughts and activities, they have a life they are involved in apart from cancer.

It is a shame that in some conventional medical environments, these patients can still be unfairly seen as 'difficult' in that they will speak up for themselves and wish to question and discuss all aspects of their treatment rather than just be told what to do and follow the 'process'.

Interview July 2011

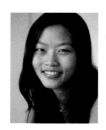

Dr Lynette Yong
MA (Cantab) FRCS

Dr Yong trained at Cambridge and Imperial College London. After qualifying she worked in hospitals in and around London to gain her Surgical Fellowship. She now practices in the private sector, which allows her to spend plenty of time with her lovely family.

Q: **As a medic, how did you feel about your friend and colleague choosing an alternative route when diagnosed with breast cancer?**

A: Well, it was difficult because there was conflict. As a doctor, I felt I had to say, we have no proven technology that you're using here, but I also felt I really had to support her in what she had decided to do. At the end of the day, I think it's more important for a patient to have the correct attitude in respect to their illness than anything else. I think that as I've got older as a person, I've seen all sorts of unlikely things happen and it's now my belief that it's a person's attitude and reaction to their circumstances which makes the most difference to the outcome. So yes, it was very difficult but I understood that at the end of the day what she really, really, needed to do was to have support for her decision and that's the way I chose to help her.

Q: **How were you able to square your orthodox medical training when faced with your friend's decision?**

A: As I said before, I thought it was most important for her to have the mental and physical support that I could give her, as a doctor. So I was able to help her with a few things. From the point of view of what she wanted, I felt it was really important that she had the sort of support that she needed and it was important for me to listen to what she needed, rather than to impose my feelings about what she should do. At the end of the day, it's really easy for us as doctors to feel that what we know is right and complete but we have so much that we don't understand and are often too afraid to admit that.

Q: **Did you try to persuade her otherwise and, if not, why not?**

A: I didn't, because I don't think she would have let me, and that would have been the end of the conversation if I'd even started. I don't think I would have seen her for a few years so, no, I didn't!

Q: **Has her personal experience influenced your own beliefs and attitudes in any way?**

A: Well, it's confirmed to me completely, that the way you think about your adversity makes a difference to your outcome. The way that you choose to express how you feel about what's happened to you, and what you then decide to do about it, is so important and the whole process of taking control, being in charge of your own illness, with the help of professionals and their expertise is really important. It's important for people not to feel like they've been victimised, because, after all, any cancer is just a group of cells in your body that has gone wrong for lots of different reasons whether it's due to exposure to toxins or a weakened immune system. We have the best tools for fighting it inside us. We have our own inbuilt immune system, so if we could harness some sort of self resurrecting power for the immune system, it would be wonderful. So, has it changed my attitudes and beliefs? No, it's confirmed what I've suspected for a long time.

Q: **What's your own medical experience of cancer treatments?**

A: I'm not a cancer specialist but, of course, during my training I've encountered many cancer patients. I trained as a surgeon, where the main modalities for removing and treating cancers were basically to cut it out. Although it wasn't always successful, it often was, which is why we continue to do it, but cancer's a difficult entity because it's not a single thing, it's a group of internal cells that have gone rogue or maverick and have decided to do things differently. There are many different causes so it's really a 'bucket theory', nobody really knows if there is a single entity which makes it occur, but we know that people can have a propensity, and based on a whole set of circumstance they might be living in, combined with their emotional state perhaps, combined with exposure to external triggers, combined with their genetic weaknesses or susceptibilities, people develop cancers.

I think to look at cancer as a single, fearful thing is not useful for anybody, patients or doctors and yet I know the word itself evokes so much fear. We must work really hard to change that, maybe by changing the word or not using the word in relation to some of the diseases which are very curable.

Q: **What do you feel may be the future of Cancer care?**

A: I think, at least I hope, that we'll move towards treating patients in a more individualistic way in allowing them to combine their beliefs if they wish to use alternative therapies, if they are compatible with what we know in modern medicine. I think our screening methods and our detection and our ability to follow a cancer, are very well established and very good. However, whilst our treatments are very good, I think they could be augmented by the use of lifestyle changes such as, diet and supplements, as well as encouraging a positive belief in the patient's ability to cure themselves. How we do this will obviously depend on each individual practitioner, physician, and surgeon as well as the patient. I think we have to find the right combination of things to make it work for a patient. Not every doctor is right for every patient. Sometimes a patient will respond very well to an authoritarian attitude as in, "I will tell you what you need to do", and some patients respond better to a more democratic environment where they're allowed to choose. I think it's important to be sensitive to that, though not possible in all cases unfortunately.

Q: **Any other comments?**

A: Well to everybody out there, Jess is living proof that you can do it!

Interview April 2011

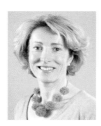

Dr Caroline Hoffman
PhD RN BSW
Clinical and Research
Director, Breast Cancer Haven.

Caroline has specialised in integrated healthcare for over 20 years both in the NHS and voluntary sector. Her last NHS role was as the first Nurse Consultant in Cancer Rehabilitation at the Royal Marsden NHS Foundation Trust. Caroline's long-standing expertise in psychosocial support, nursing and complementary therapies enables her to lead the teams of specialist nurses, therapists and researchers across all Havens. For her PhD she evaluated the effectiveness of a Mindfulness-Based Stress Reduction (MBSR) programme in a randomised controlled trial of 229 women who had been treated for breast cancer and attended The Haven. This rigorous study produced very positive results. She continues to teach MBSR at The Haven in London. These courses are open to all.

Caroline is also a member of the following national committees: The National Cancer Research Institute Complementary Therapies Clinical Studies Development Group; and the Editorial Board of NHS Evidence – Complementary and Alternative Medicine. She has also been active in contributing to the National Cancer Survivorship Initiative to help develop the national strategy for improving the lives of people living with cancer.

Q: **What inspired you to practice at the Breast Cancer Haven?**

A: I started to work at the Haven, helping to develop the service here when the charity started. I had been working with integrated medicine for a number of years. I started using integrated medicine in the intensive setting at the Middlesex Hospital where

I did some research, and later at the Hospital that is now known as 'The London Hospital for Integrated Medicine' where I was part of the complimentary cancer clinic. So my own background is in psychology and social work, I'm a nurse and I've specialised in a range of complimentary therapies. And I completed my PHD evaluating mindfulness-based stress reduction in people affected by breast cancer.

Q: **Have you noticed any changes in the treatment choices of cancer patients?**

A: There's a growing interest amongst patients about how they can help themselves, and I think there's growing awareness of the more recent initiatives, such as the National Cancer Survivorship Initiative. There's a growing interest into how people can contribute to their own health and wellbeing. I think the days are long gone where people want to rely solely on what is done at the hospital, because they want to take an active part in their own recovery. I think this is very important because we are all responsible for our own health and wellbeing in the long run. We may not be able to cure ourselves, but we can make a substantial contribution to improving and sustaining good health even in the face of a major illness.

Q: **Have patients' attitudes towards treatments changed over the years and if so, how?**

A: In terms of the treatments breast cancer patients choose, in my experience of working with people with cancer in an integrated setting for 20 years, there has always been a percentage of people who are seeking to use the diagnosis as a springboard for their own development of their health and wellbeing. This is not only in terms of improvement of physical health and wellbeing, but also psychological, emotional, and mental health and wellbeing. What bigger wake-up call could there possibly be in life than the diagnosis of cancer? Diagnosis of cancer or any major illness gives us the opportunity to look at our lives and see what it is that we could do better or more skilfully to enhance our own health and happiness.

Q: **Has your attitude changed over the years and if so, how?**

A: As I've got older, I guess, at least I hope I've got a little wiser! But that could be up for debate. I think that working with people with life-threatening illness for many years, and also looking at the way I need to work with my own health and wellbeing, we learn from our own experience. I think to be good practitioners, we need to be walking our talk. We have to be actively engaged in processes that help our mental, emotional, physical and social development and wellbeing otherwise I don't believe that we can be good with other people. Unless we demonstrate our own thing, how can we possibly help other people grow as well. So my attitude has probably grown in the sense that I've grown in understanding of what it's like to be a human being and what factors can affect our health and wellbeing.

Also, as time's gone on there are many more resources becoming available that can help people, so when faced with something like a diagnosis of cancer, there are many more options available to tap into. I think that one of the things about the Haven is that we offer a wide range of resources very deliberately, because what suits one person may not suit another. We have to be able to cater for the needs of people in a variety of ways to serve both mind and body and also provide energy therapies, healing, practical things like nutritional advice and acupuncture and so on. We also consider psychological approaches, the mind /body approaches, things like mindfulness, meditation, counselling, and mind/body work in general.

All these things have a really vital contribution to make and some will appeal to some people and some to others, and at different stages. Maybe some will start with one kind of treatment and then move on when something else opens up and they feel it's appropriate to take on some other kind

Q: **Have you noticed any changes in attitudes from consultants and other medics?**

A: I think that there are many medical, nursing and other people working in hospitals who are now much more open to other options. They're open to the idea of how people can help themselves. Anyone with any wisdom can see that medical treatment is only part of the answer and I think any wise medical consultant or cancer specialist can see that they're working as part of a larger team which includes the patient, themselves and all the other people who are working to help the person who is facing the illness.

I think there are a lot of people who are now much more interested. As consultants get older they may think that they've got more answers, and I think that as they get older they see things from a wider perspective. I think there are many wonderful doctors out there who are very willing to support people in the way they would want to be supported themselves. If a patient finds him or herself in a place where they're not with somebody who understands that, maybe they should ask around and find the right person or team.

Q: **What is your experience of cancer professionally or personally?**

A: Professionally, I came to working with people with cancer as a MacMillan clinical nurse specialist in complementary therapies in the early 1990s. I had virtually no personal experience of it at that stage. Since that time, both my sister and my sister-in-law have been diagnosed and treated for breast cancer so I now have a close association with it from that point of view. I had a serious illness (not cancer) myself when I was younger, at university, and that lay the foundations for me to look at life and at health and wellbeing with a different view. I know the things that helped me then are still helping to keep me well now. So it's not about being a one-way-street, we have some responsibility to maintain our health and wellbeing rather than waiting until something goes wrong and then expecting other people to fix it.

Q: **What is the first thing you would advise someone to do on receiving a cancer diagnosis?**

A: The wise thing would be for them to stop and pause for a moment and to take stock but that's very easy to say and incredibly difficult to do because the minute that somebody's diagnosed, as we know, they're immediately thrown into this situation of total shock. Their whole world is turned upside down and they're expected to make very complex treatment decisions in a very short period of time. So I think that the first thing I would say is have good people around you and take time to listen to what's being said. Make sure that you're happy, in that you understand what's happening and what's being said to you and if you're not sure then don't feel pushed into doing something immediately. With most breast cancer diagnosis, things can wait a bit in that it's not an emergency where things have to be done in a matter of a few days or even a few weeks. Things can wait.

I think people don't realise that they can take time to explore and make sure that they are really happy with the decisions they've made. There is time to talk to people such as staff at the Haven, or seek out advice from other specialists who can support them in making those decisions. It doesn't have to be done in a hurry unless the doctor has indicated the situation is a medical emergency. Taking your time will not make any detrimental difference to the outcome. It's more important to do what's right for you.

Q: **What, in your experience is the most common factor in those who survive cancer?**

A: Now this gets me onto an interesting topic. I'm going to start at the other end of this question if I may. The first thing I want to say is that we don't know why anybody gets any illness in the first place. We have our genetic make-up, we have our nature, we have our nurture we have our environment, we have our whole upbringing. We have the physical and emotional impact of that, we have all those factors. We've also got the life we've led up until the point that something happens with our health. In my view, all those things have contributed to whatever breakdown in health we have whether it's physical or mental. Something goes wrong that is the product of where we've got up to in our lives.

So we have to start where we are, wherever that happens to be and for everybody, it will be different. I think that we have our own individual ways of working through what those priorities are, what we do and when, what we choose to look at, and what we choose to get help with.

Often in the early stage of being diagnosed, we need just to stop, we need to be held, we need to be in this kind of safe container where we have a chance to take a while to work out what's important to us and then, when we've been able to let the dust settle a little bit, when there's a chance to raise our head above the parapet and take a step back to take a bigger view, then we can start to make decisions about the steps we should take as individuals that will help our situation.

I don't believe that there is any one particular thing that everybody has to do, I believe it differs from person to person. For some people it will be more physical, help with diet or exercise, whereas with others it may be mental or emotional or spiritual help that will be the priority. We must consider whether we can calm ourselves or get help to calm down so that we can be in a state where we can listen to some of those inner needs.

So, in answer to the question, what is the most common factor, I would say there is a willingness on the part of the person to work with themselves in whatever way is necessary.

Q: What would you advise as a long term survival strategy?

A: This comes back to the last question in that we have got to get to know ourselves and we've got to get to know the things that help us and what works for us. What are the things that bring us more ease, relaxation, vitality, health and wellbeing and joy into our own lives? How can we create that? Can we be honest with ourselves? In order to improve our health and wellbeing in any way, we have got to be authentic. We must ask ourselves what it is that we need and to start from that basis.

Q: What do you feel is the future of cancer treatment?

A: I think the future of cancer treatment is individualised. If we're talking about medical treatment it's individualised! It won't be a mass approach because we're learning more and more that each cancer with each person is different, and in terms of medical technology, if we can see what the individuals need we can treat each individual cancer differently.

Also, for many years now I've been talking about an integrated approach. Looking at the mind and the body together. We're not going to crack health, happiness and wellbeing by just going down one narrow route, we have to look at the wider picture.

Q: Anything else you would like to add?

A: Yes, I'd like to talk about the Haven.

The Breast Cancer Haven is a registered charity that is set up to provide free help and support to anyone affected by breast cancer. This support is in addition to any hospital treatment to enhance the individual's health and wellbeing and the quality of life for anybody going through a breast cancer experience. Our ethos is that no-one should face breast cancer alone, because people often need a lot of help and support around them and more importantly the right kind of help and support. Sometimes family and friends mean very well but they don't know how to help. So we're here for people so they can access professional advice in a beautiful healing environment which is nurturing, and where they can learn ways to help themselves.

Interview September 2011

Recommended reading

There are many worthwhile books out there but I've created this short list of those I've read and found to be particularly helpful.

Getting Well Again
Carl Simonton MD,
Stephanie Matthews-Simonton
and James Creighton
ISBN 0-87477-070-X

Cancer As a Turning Point
Lawrence LeShan PhD
ISBN 0-525-24743-2

Remarkable Recovery
Caryle Hirshberg
and Marc Ian Barasch
ISBN 0-7472-4813-3

Take Control Of Your Health
Dr Joseph Mercola
and Dr Kendra Pearsall
Available from www.mercola.com

How To Achieve Healthy Aging
Neal Rouzier, MD
ISBN 0-9710007-3-5

Reinventing Medicine
Larry Dossey, MD
ISBN 0-06-251622-1

Recovering the Soul
Larry Dossey MD
ISBN 0-553-34790-X

Healing Words
Larry Dossey MD
ISBN 0-06-250252-2

The Extraordinary Healing Power of Ordinary Things
Larry Dossey MD
ISBN 978-0-307-20990-0

The Power Of Premonitions
Larry Dossey MD
ISBN 978-1-8485-0166-9

The Science of Premonition
Larry Dossey MD
ISBN 978-0-525-95116-2

Healing Beyond the Body
Larry Dossey MD
ISBN 978-0-7499-2994-7

Be Careful What You Pray For
Larry Dossey MD
ISBN 0-06-251433-4

The Essential Guide to Water and Salt
F. Batmanghelidj, MD and Phillip Day
ISBN 1-904015-22-0

Health Wars
Phillip Day
ISBN 0-9535012-7-2

Cancer: Why We're Still Dying to Know The Truth
Phillip Day
ISBN 0-0953512-4-8

Simple Changes
Phillip Day
ISBN 1-904015-20-4

The Power of Now
Eckhart Tolle
ISBN 978-0-340-73350-9

Practising the Power of Now
Eckhart Tolle
ISBN 978-0-340-82253-1

When Everything Changes Change Everything
Neale Donald Walsch
ISBN 978-1-57174-606-1

The Biology of Belief
Bruce H. Lipton, PhD
ISBN 978-1-4019-2311-2

The Hidden Power for HumanProblems
Frederick Bailes
ISBN 57-13274

Your Mind Can Heal You
Frederick Bailes
ISBN 087516-201-07

Living Proof
Michael Gearin-Tosh
ISBN 0-7432-0680-0

Loving What Is
Byron Katie
ISBN 0-7126-2930-0

The German New Medicine
Dr Hamer
Available from www.newmedia.ca

The Miracle of Mind Power
Dan Custer
ISBN 0-930298-20-9

Everything you Need to Know To Help You Beat Cancer
Chris Woollams
ISBN 0-9542968-5-0

Useful resources

World Cancer Research Fund
www.wcrf-uk.org *(charity)*

Breast Cancer Haven
www.thehaven.org.uk *(charity)*

Vision of Hope Clinic
www.visionofhopeclinic.com

Phillip Day
www.campaignfortruth.com

Dr Mercola
www.mercola.com

Icon / Cancer Active
www.canceractive.com *(charity)*

Dr Hamer (The German New Medicine)
www.newmedicine.ca

Brightspot.org
www.brightspot.org *(charity)*

Cancer Options (Patricia Peat)
www.canceroptions.co.uk

Yes to Life
www.yestolife.org.uk *(charity)*

The Holly Eatwell trust
www.thehollyeatwelltrust.com *(charity)*

iHealthtube
www.ihealthtube.com

Acknowledgements

I would like to acknowledge and express my sincere and heartfelt Thanks to the many people and organisations who have helped me with their prayers, thoughts, words and deeds and especially to the following people for their, love, support and expertise:

My late Father Chuck, for never doubting my ability to make the right decisions and never questioning my judgement.

My late mother Kathleen, for somehow remaining strong for me throughout the agonies of your own situation and your fears for mine.

Alan Boxall the giant beside me on the road to hell.

Mr Mark Kissin for your professional experience and expertise and especially your patience, respect, support and humanity.

Dr Andre Young Snell for your professional support and dedication and for your ability to make the experience fun whenever possible.

Sheila, Alan's mum, for your loving care and support especially in the early days of treatment when you cared for me in your home as one of your own.

The late Gil Boyne: 28.9.1924 - 5.5.2010. My American 'Father'. Thank you for being my teacher and mentor, and for believing in me all those years ago.

My friend Marisa Peer for accompanying me and watching over me like a guardian angel.

Dr Lynette Yong for your loyal and loving friendship, support and professionalism.

Brenda Golding for your constant loving support and professional expertise.

Joanna Jesson for your love and friendship and for diligently conveying the information to our professional colleagues.

Andy Lowe, for keeping me supplied with all the weird and wonderful supplements I needed at a very generous discount which helped enable me to buy what I needed rather than what I could afford.

Paul and Kate Ugo for keeping me supplied with your excellent Chickpea pasta.

Josef and Krystina Pajes for your love and practical support.

The 'Harley Gang' Roy Jones, Tim Hancock and Steve Feery for your friendship, support and practical input.

Phillip Day for your patient support and invaluable research material which helped me to make informed decisions.

My GP, Dr Jackson, for your support and patience in the early days, and for not losing your nerve!

Patricia Peat for your information, experience and support.

Peter Pritchett ACE Chairman for your friendship as well as professional and moral support. Thank you also to the other members of group DF2.

The "Fabulous Womens' Group" Andrea, Deborah, Joanna, Lisa, Julia and Mandy for all your love, laughter and support and for making me finish this book.

My extraordinarily talented professional team

Victoria Barry, my editor, for your honesty, enthusiasm and professionalism. victoria@red-carpet.co.uk

Neil Kerber for your support and the brilliant cartoons in this book. neil@neilkerber.com

Thank you to Luby for the great photos. markloo63@yahoo.co.uk

Brigitte Whitefield, design and layout. brigitte@b-created.com

Richard Painter, print production. info@printresources.co.uk

And charities Breast Cancer Haven and Yes to Life for your invaluable help and support.

My Team

Well, you've read about some of my team members in this book and I thought you might like to put the lovely faces to the names - Ta da!

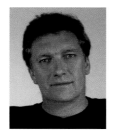

Alan

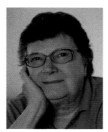

Sheila

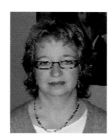

Brenda

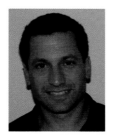

Andy

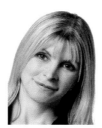

Marisa

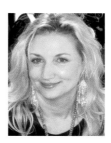

Astrid

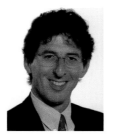

Mr Mark Kissin

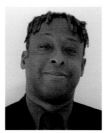

Dr Andre Young-Snell

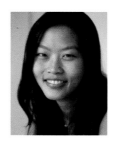

Dr Lynette Yong

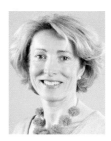

Dr Caroline Hoffman

Notes

Notes

Notes

Notes

Notes

Notes

Notes

Notes

Notes

Notes